The Keto for Two Cookbook:

550 Low-Carb Recipes to Lose Weight and Feel Great

Copyright © 2020 Helena Ortiz

All rights reserved. No part of this publication may be reproduced or distributed in any form or by any means, electronic or mechanical, photocopying, scanning, recording or otherwise, without prior written permission from the publisher and the author.

Disclaimer of Warranty / Limit of Liability: The author and the publisher are not a licensed physician, medical professional or practitioner and offers no medical counseling, treatments or diagnoses. The author and the publisher make no warranties with respect to the accuracy and completeness of the contents of this work. All the nutritional facts contained in this book is provided for informational purposes only. The information is based on the specific ingredients, measurements and brands used to make the recipe. Therefore, the nutritional facts in this work in no way is intended to be a guarantee of the actual nutritional value of the recipe made by the reader. The author and the publisher will not be responsible for any damages resulting in reliance of the reader on the nutritional information.

The content presented herein, has not been evaluated by the U.S. Food and Drug Administration, and it is not intended to cure or diagnose any disease. This book isn't intended as a substitute for medical advice as physicians. Full medical clearance from a licensed physician should be obtained before beginning any diet. The advice and strategies contained herein may not be suitable for every situation. Neither the author nor the publisher claims no responsibility to any person or entity for any liability, damage or loss caused directly or indirectly as a result of the use, application or interpretation of the information presented in this work.

The publisher publishes its books in a variety of print and electronic formats. Some content that appears in print may not be available in electronic, and vice versa.

Table of Contents

Introduction 7
Ketogenic Breakfast Recipes 8
- Radish Hash 8
- Kale Eggs 8
- Vanilla Bowls 8
- Chia Pudding 8
- Rosemary Porridge 8
- Stevia and Nuts Bowls 8
- Cinnamon Bowls 8
- Blackberries Salad 8
- Scallions Eggs 9
- Red Pepper Flakes Eggs 9
- White Mushroom and Cumin Eggs 9
- Green Avocado Salad 9
- Almonds and Berries Bowls 9
- Lime Zest Salad 9
- Salmon and Cumin Eggs 9
- Shallot Salad 9
- Avocado Smoothie 10
- Ginger Smoothie 10
- Micro Greens Bowls 10
- Sweet Paprika Eggs Mix 10
- Nuts Bowls 10
- Sweet Avocado Salad 10
- Seafood and Parsley Bowls 10
- Coconut Eggs 10
- Hard Boiled Eggs Bowl 11
- Garlic Shrimps Mix 11
- Salmon Salad 11
- Black Olives Salad 11
- Cheese and Turkey Mix 11
- Keto Passata 11
- Chives, Spinach, and Shrimps 11
- Keto Vegetables and Beef Stew 12
- Basil and Shrimps Salad 12
- Cilantro Pork Meatballs 12
- Coconut Cream Soup 12
- Keto Style Mix 12
- Soft Meatballs 12
- Rosemary Broccoli with Beef 13
- Tender Tuna Mix 13
- Aromatic Beef and Greens 13
- Keto Radish Salad 13
- Mushrooms and Pork 13
- Turkey and Endives 13
- Dill Fritters 14
- Stew Meat Bowls 14
- Cilantro and Eggs Mix 14
- Green Spread 14
- Oregano and Tuna Casserole 14
- Parmesan Eggs Mix 14
- Garam Masala Meal 15
- Green Beans with Chicken 15
- Keto Cheese Mix 15
- Salmon Stew 15
- Garlic Mix 15
- Meat Casserole 15
- Spiced Meat Stew 16
- Basil and Seafood Bowls 16
- Cabbage Soup 16
- Kale and Garlic Soup 16
- Poultry and Fish Soup 16
- Meat and Spinach Bowls 16
- Jalapeno Chicken Thighs 17
- Walnuts and Beef Bowl 17
- Baby Spinach and Avocado Salad 17
- Almond Pancakes 17
- Turmeric Pancakes 17
- Garlic Zucchini 17
- Onion Powder Eggs 18
- Hot Eggs 18
- Cheddar Cheese Bake 18
- Spinach Bowl 18
- Green Lime Omelet 18
- Capers and Tuna Salad 18
- Poultry and Cucumber Salad 18
- Turmeric Sprouts Soup 19
- Spiralized Salad 19
- Spiced Chicken Pan 19
- Cream and Cauliflower Soup 19
- Chicken Pan 19
- Chicken Sauce 19
- Crab Mix 20
- Salmon and Capers Salad 20
- Vinegar Shrimps 20
- Lunch Shrimps 20
- Cherry Tomatoes and Shrimps Bowl 20
- Turmeric Eggs with Shrimps 20
- Chives Muffins 20
- Ghee Eggs Mix 21
- Lime Juice and Poultry Salad 21
- Almond and Coconut Porridge Bowls 21
- Sweet Omelet 21
- Turmeric Brussels Sprouts 21
- Basil Salad 21
- Baby Spinach and Chicken Bowls 21
- Baby Spinach Soup 21
- Chili Powder Meat 22
- Poultry Stew 22
- Turkey Stew 22
- Aromatic Basil Shrimps 22
- Parsley Fish Stew 22
- Curry Turkey 22
- Parsley Soup 23
- Passata Soup 23
- White Mushrooms Stew 23
- Minced Garlic and Scallions Beef 23
- Capers Mix 23
- Ground Beef Bowl 23
- Lime Juice and Chives Salad 24
- Avocado and Eggs 24
- Ilspice Zucchini 24
- Almond and Vegetables Muffins 24
- Ketogenic Lunch Recipes 24
- Scallions and Seafood Salad 24
- Morning Waffles 25
- Paprika Chicken Thighs 25
- Kalamata and Chicken Salad 25
- Tender Keto Muffins 25
- Green Onions Shrimp 25
- Chili Pepper Soup 25
- Mix of Seeds Bowls 26
- Bell Peppers Scrambled Eggs 26
- Garlic Frittata 26
- Cilantro Eggs 26
- Shrimps and Vegetables 26
- Bell Peppers Saute 26
- Cucumbers and Olives Salad 27
- Arugula Salad 27
- White Mushrooms and Lamb Mix 27
- Walnuts Salad 27
- Lemon Seabass with Avocado 27

Ketogenic Side Dish Recipes 28
- Basil Salad 28
- Salad with Lime Juice 28
- Paprika Asparagus 28
- Spring Onions Salad 28
- Kale Saute 28
- Radish and Cabbage 28
- Chives Cauliflower 28
- Scallions Zucchini 28
- Baby Spinach Saute 29
- Marinated Cucumbers 29
- Cumin Stew 29
- Lime Taste Salad 29

Sliced Cucumbers and Cabbage Salad 29
Dill Zoodles 29
Fennel Bulb Salad 29
Keto Avocado Bowl 29
Flaked Red Pepper Mushrooms 30
Zucchini Medley 30
Hemp Seeds Mushrooms 30
Spiced Vegetables 30
Green Chili Pepper Tomatoes 30
Sage Zucchini 30
Lime and Vinegar Cauliflower 30
Tender Zucchini Rice 31
Mustard Seeds Kale 31
Tarragon Fennel 31
Tender Radish Stew 31
Classic Keto Bowl 31
Cayenne Pepper Cauli 31
Rosemary Peppers 32
Mustard Greens and Olives 32
Baby Arugula Salad 32
Fragrant Scallions 32
Dill and Cucumber Bowl 32
Green Mushrooms 32
Hot Cauli Rice 32
Tender Red Cabbage 32
Aromatic Keto Mix 33
Herbs de Provence Olives 33
Jalapeno and Cheddar Cheese Mix 33
Soft and Aromatic Radish Bowl 33
Cumin and Oregano Radish 33
Indian Style Cauliflower 33
Rosemary Mushroom Rice 33
Coconut Cream and Cumin Radish Mix 34
Cumin Kale 34
Aromatic Brussel Sprouts 34
Fragrant Mushrooms 34
Cumin Green Beans 34
Parmesan Radishes 34
Kalamata Olives and Fennel 35
Dill Mix 35
Dijon Mustard Mix 35
Keto Caps 35
Chili Powder Salad 35
Tender Ghee Rice 35
Cilantro and Vegetables Mix 36
Cajun Seasonings and Keto Vegetables 36
Herbs de Provence Olives 36
Caraway Seeds Mix of Vegetables 36
Chives Stew 36

Ketogenic Snacks and Appetizers Recipes 37

Parsley Cheese Spread 37
Mozzarella and Vegetables Dip 37
Kale and Scallions Salsa 37
Seeds and Nuts Snack 37
Ketogenic Seafood and Fish Recipes 37
Meat Muffins 37
Turmeric Trout 37
Oregano Dip 37
Garlic Sea Bass 38
Lime Salmon 38
Tender Lemon Shrimp 38
Shrimps with Chicken broth 38
Radish Dip 38
Walnuts Dip 38
Pesto and Zucchini Dip 38
Walnuts Snack Bowls 38
Lime Cream Dip 39
Smoked Shrimp Platter 39
Broccoli Bites 39
Masala Dip 39
Peppers Salsa 39
Seeds Snack 39
Olives and Cream Cheese Spread 39
Cucumbers Salsa 39
Ghee and Garlic Spread 40
Spring Onions Chicken Bites 40
Nutmeg Platter 40
Poblano Peppers Dip 40
Cheese Sticks 40
Capers Salsa 40
Lamb and Garlic Dip 40
Mint Spread 40
Dijon Mustard Trout 41
Paprika Zucchini Chips 41
Keto Salsa 41
Green Dip 41
Basil Pesto Dip 41
Coconut Cream Dip 41
Cilantro Sea Bass 41
Scallions Shrimps 41
Sun Dried Tomatoes and Olives Salsa 42
Avocado Dip 42
Cumin Bowls 42
Asparagus and Lime Zest Bowls 42
Garlic Wings 42
Greens and Capers Salad 42
Chives Salsa 42
Cucumber and Dill Dip 42
Salmon Mix 43
Keto Eggs Salad 43
Dijon Shrimp Skewers 43
Keto Vegetables Rolls 43
Fennel Seeds Shrimp 43
Parsley and Shrimps Bowl 43
Ginger Tuna 43
Scallions Dip 44
Balsamic Tuna with Spring Onions 44
Nutmeg Salmon Bowl 44
Garlic Powder Dip 44
Spring Onions Dip 44
Vegetable Spread 44
Coconut Muffins 44
Cheese Dip 45
Chicken Muffins 45
Seafood Meatballs 45
Fish Platter 45
Kale and Parsley Dip 45
Shrimp and Curry Powder Salsa 45
Italian Style Shrimps 45
Basil Tuna and Cayenne Pepper Bowl 46
Turmeric Calamari 46
Calamari with Zucchini Zoodles 46
Shrimps with Fresh Fennel Bulb 46
Shrimps with Endives 46
Baby Spinach and Fish Salad 46
Pesto Snack 47
Curry and Garlic Shrimps 47
Cod with Coriander Sauce 47
Sour Cumin Shrimp 47
Chia and Flaxseeds Muffins 47
Avocado Mix with Calamari Rings 47
Red Pepper Flakes Trout 48
Cauli and Shrimps 48
Shrimps in Sauce 48
Shrimps with Green Beans 48
Chili Cod 48
Shrimps with Almonds and Parmesan 48
Rosemary Sea Bass 49
Trout Bowl 49
Oregano and Chili Cod 49
Artichoke and Parmesan Spread 49
Rosemary and Chives Salmon 49
Coriander Calamari with Olives 49
Green Onions Calamari 50
Aromatic Shrimps with Pine Nuts 50
Coconut Milk Cod 50
Coriander Cod 50
Avocado with Cod 50
Tuna with Vegetables 50

Tender Salmon with Ghee ... 51
Ginger and Cumin Salmon ... 51
Vegetables with Calamari ... 51
Tender Sour Tuna ... 51
Coconut Cream Shrimps ... 51
Perfect Keto Tuna ... 51
Shrimps and Bell Peppers Bowl ... 52
Aromatic Trout ... 52
Fish with Mustard Sauce ... 52
Salmon with Halved Tomatoes ... 52
Thyme Seafood Bowl ... 52
Marjoram Seafood Bowl ... 52
Garlic Mussels ... 53
Tarragon and Cumin Swordfish Steaks ... 53
Baked Cod with Parsley ... 53
Sea Bass and Baby Kale Bowl ... 53
Tender Fish and Cabbage Salad ... 53
Spiced Tuna Fillets ... 53
Keto Crackers ... 54
Chili Dip ... 54
Mint and Garlic Shrimp ... 54

Ketogenic Poultry Recipes ... 55

Turmeric Chicken ... 55
Coriander Turkey Bowl ... 55
Tender Chicken Cubes with Kalamata Olives ... 55
Chicken with Curry Paste and Coconut Cream ... 55
Poultry Stir Fry ... 55
Rosemary Chicken with Artichokes ... 55
Tender Chicken and Greens ... 56
Herbs and Chicken Mix ... 56
Shredded Cabbage and Chicken Mix ... 56
Garam Masala Chicken ... 56
Oregano Turkey ... 56
Red Chili Pepper Turkey ... 56
Zucchini and Ground Chicken Bowl ... 57
Leek and Turkey ... 57
Coriander Chicken with Fennel ... 57
Cauliflower Florets with Ginger Chicken ... 57
Cumin and Coconut Cream Chicken Breast ... 57
Sesame and Ginger Chicken ... 57
Vegetables and Chicken Strips ... 58
Green Beans and Turkey ... 58
Cheddar Chicken Thighs ... 58
Mustard and Garlic Chicken ... 58
Basil and Garlic Chicken ... 58
Chicken with Endives ... 58
Bella Mushrooms and Turkey ... 59
Chicken in Tender Sauce ... 59
Parmesan Chicken with Radish ... 59
Chicken Roast ... 59
Garam Masala Duck ... 59
Lemon Turkey Bowl ... 59
Mushrooms, Parsley, and Chicken Bowl ... 60
Broccoli and Poultry Bowl ... 60
Spicy Chicken Breast Cubes ... 60
Chives Chicken ... 60
Mozzarella Chicken ... 60
Ghee and Parmesan Chicken ... 60
Cheese Chicken ... 61
Scallions Chicken Cubes ... 61
Radish Halves with Chicken Cubes ... 61
Garlic Turkey Breast with Brussels Sprouts ... 61
Aromatic Spiced Turkey ... 61
Nutmeg Chicken Cubes ... 61
Asparagus and Tender Chicken Thighs ... 62
Rosemary and Paprika Chicken ... 62
Poultry Bake ... 62
Greens and Turkey Bowl ... 62
Tender Turkey in Sauce ... 62
Lime Zest Chicken ... 62
Chili Powder Turkey ... 63
Fragrant Cumin Turkey ... 63
Poultry and Spinach Mix ... 63
Salsa Verde Turkey ... 63
Cilantro Chicken ... 63
Chicken with Artichokes ... 63
Hot Chicken ... 64
Chicken and Leek Bowl ... 64
Thyme Chicken ... 64
Tender Duck ... 64
Mustard Powder Turkey ... 64
Chili Chicken Wings ... 64

Ketogenic Meat Recipes ... 65

Pork and Zucchini ... 65
Parmesan Meat ... 65
Tender Lamb with Ghee ... 65
Cheesy Cumin and Garlic Beef ... 65
Autumn Beef Mix ... 65
Nutmeg Pork Cubes ... 65
Beef and Peppers ... 66
Pork and Cauli Mix ... 66
Coriander Meat Stew ... 66
Juicy Rosemary Pork ... 66
Garlic Mushroom with Bok Choy ... 66
Chives and Avocado Mix ... 66
Spring Pork Stew ... 67
Spicy Okra and Beef Bowl ... 67
Keto Meat with Vegetables ... 67
Pork with Coriander and Shredded Cabbage ... 67
Aromatic Parsley and Lamb Stew ... 67
Cumin and Bell Pepper Pork ... 67
Chives Radishes ... 68
Rosemary Tomatoes ... 68
Chili Fennel ... 68
Garlic and Chives Asparagus ... 68
Olives and Scallions Salad ... 68
Spring Salad ... 68
Baby Kale Mix ... 68
Cilantro Avocado ... 68
Cherry Tomatoes and Greens Salad ... 69
Paprika and Lime Bok Choy ... 69
Broccoli Florets Bowl ... 69
Zucchini Cubes Stew ... 69
Asparagus Stew ... 69
Cheesy Artichokes ... 69
Basil Green Beans ... 69
Sprouts and Kale Bowl ... 69
Greens Bowl ... 70
Coconut Cream Bok Choy ... 70
Black Pepper Radishes ... 70
Baby Kale and Halved Radish ... 70
Keto Broccoli Mix ... 70
Basil Cream ... 70
Coconut Cream Zucchini ... 70
Chili and Chives Lamb ... 71
Scallions and Celery Stalk Lamb ... 71
Keto Lamb Bowl ... 71
Pork Chops with Vegetables ... 71
Green Beans with Chili Pork ... 71
Chili Peppers Lamb Chops ... 71
Dill and Cayenne Pepper Beef ... 72
Meat Salad with Capers ... 72
Vinegar Beef ... 72
Parsley Lamb Cubes ... 72
Mint Lamb Cubes ... 72
Garlic Cubed Pork ... 72
Scallions Lamb Chops ... 73
Ketogenic Vegetable Recipes ... 73
Cilantro Brussels Sprouts ... 73
Tender Beef Roast ... 73
Italian Seasoning and Pesto Lamb ... 73
Radish and Lamb Stew ... 73
Chili Powder Pork Stew Meat ... 74
Parmesan and Scallions Lamb Chops ... 74
Lamb with Capers ... 74
Walnuts Salad ... 74
Tender Keto Salad ... 74
Turmeric Sliced Zucchini Mix ... 74

Table of Contents | 5

Pork with Sliced Fennel 74
Garlic Peppers 75
Garam Masala Green Cabbage 75
Broccoli Spread 75
Cumin Swiss Chard with Kalamata Olives 75
Tender Cilantro Lamb Chops 75
Garam Masala Brussels Sprouts 75
Garam Masala Beef with Artichokes 76
Cumin and Chili Powder Lamb Chops 76
Kale and Ground Beef 76
Turmeric Bok Choy 76
Garam Masala Lamb 76
Coconut Cream Beef 76
Ginger and Rosemary Broccoli 77
Passata Pork Chops 77
Tender Sour Lamb Riblets 77
Tomato Passata Kale 77
Rosemary Lamb 77
Cumin Cauliflower 77
Coconut Aminos Pork 78
Cumin Pork Chops 78
Rosemary Beef with Swiss Chard 78
Chili Lamb with Mushrooms 78
Rosemary Pork Cubes 78
Cumin Pork with Avocado 78
Chili Beef with Tarragon 79
Dill Mix 79
Aromatic Lamb Chops 79
Tender Beef Stew Meat 79
Fennel Mix 79
Creamy Sprouts 79
Lemon and Coriander Brussels Sprouts 80
Red Chili Baby Spinach 80
Rosemary Green Beans 80
Sesame and Coriander Kale 80
Cubed Avocado and Pork 80
Cilantro Swiss Chard 80
Nutmeg Cauliflower 80
Lime Juice Lamb Chops 81
Succulent Beef 81
Rosemary Sprouts with Avocado 81
Lemon Lamb 81
Garlic Okra 81
Baby Spinach Bowl 81
Cabbage and Scallions 81
Keto Vegetables Stew 82
Oregano Endives 82
Soft Ghee Lamb 82
Garlic and Scallions Bok Choy 82
Chard Bowl 82
Mustard and Thyme Lamb Leg 82

Ketogenic Dessert Recipes 83
Stevia Cream 83
Heavy Cream Mix 83
Berries Mix 83
Ginger Bowls 83
Ginger Cookies 83
Swerve and Watermelon Mix 83
Ghee and Mint Cookies 83
Vanilla and Berries Bowls 84
Plums Mix 84
Plum and Vanilla Bowls 84
Mint and Watermelon Salad 84
Lime Mousse 84
Coconut and Lime Zest Custard 84
Aromatic Blueberries Mousse 84
Berries and Nutmeg Cream 84
Walnuts and Avocado Bowls 84
Cream Cheese Cream 84
Chia and Coconut Milk Pudding 85
Watermelon Soup 85
Cherries and Ginger Bowls 85
Green Tea Drink 85
Lime and Stevia Mix 85

Vanilla Fudge 85
Berry Stew 85
Delicious Keto Smoothie 85
Coconut and Cinnamon Bars 85
Cocoa and Chia Bowl 86
Berry Pie 86
Almond and Rice Pudding 86
Watermelon Custard 86
Cinnamon Pudding 86
Blackberries Salad 86
Cauliflower Pudding 86
Coconut and Cocoa Balls 86
Strawberry and Lime Saute 87
Lime Mix 87
Cream Cheese Pudding 87
Cinnamon and Vanilla Balls 87
Keto Cocoa Cream 87
Almond Cream 87
Blueberries Mousse 87
Sweet Cauli Rice 87
Avocado and Vanilla Cakes 88
Coffee Mousse 88
Zucchini Mousse 88
Avocado Mix 88
Cherry and Lemon Cream 88
Sweet and Sour Mousse 88
Nutmeg Berries Bowl 88
Keto Cheesecakes 88
Seeds Mix 89
Berries Saute 89
Almond and Berries Muffins 89
 Coconut Cream Cookies 89
Tender Avocado Pudding 89
Cocoa Powder Mix 89
Sweet and Sour Jam 89
Ghee Cupcakes 89

Recipe Index 90

Introduction

If you are searching for a healthy way to live and to lose some weight, then you should check out this great guide we developed for you.

This journal focuses on the best and most popular diet these days: the Ketogenic diet. This lifestyle will improve your appearance and your overall health in a matter of days as long as you follow its principles and you eat what you are allowed.

The Ketogenic diet is a low carb and high fat one that allows your body to enter a ketosis state. You will produce less insulin and glucose, you will soon adapt to these changes and you will begin to lose weight. You will look and feel healthier, your energy levels will increase and your mental performance as well.

The Ketogenic diet will also prevent the appearance of multiple diseases such as diabetes, heart related diseases and even epilepsy.

This diet is easy to follow and it's a lot less restrictive than many others but if you decide to follow it, you should know what you can and can not eat.

If you are on a keto diet, you can consume as many greens as you like. You can eat eggs, above ground veggies, fish, seafood, meat, poultry, nuts, seeds, healthy oils such as avocado, coconut and olive oil, avocados, berries, cheese, ghee, and cream cheese.

On the other hand, you are no longer eat grains, most fruits, sugar, beans, potatoes, yams or honey.

The Ketogenic diet recipes collection we developed for you, contains 550 of the best keto recipes for 2.

You can make some great breakfasts, lunch dishes, side dishes, appetizers, fish and seafood meals, meat, poultry and vegetable ones but also some tasty desserts for you and your loved one.

So, what are you still waiting for? Get your hands on a copy of the Ketogenic cooking guide and learn how to prepare some rich and flavored meals for 2.

Have fun and enjoy cooking some amazing Ketogenic dishes for 2!

Ketogenic Breakfast Recipes

Radish Hash

Prep time: 10 minutes | **Cooking time:** 16 minutes | **Servings:** 2

Ingredients:

- 1 tablespoon olive oil
- 2 scallions, chopped
- 4 eggs, whisked
- ¼ pound radishes, halved
- 2 garlic cloves, minced
- Salt and black pepper to the taste
- 1 tablespoon chives, chopped

Directions:

1. Heat up a pan with the oil over medium high heat, add the scallions and garlic and cook for 3 minutes.
2. Add the radishes and cook them for 3 minutes more.
3. Add the rest of the ingredients, toss, cook for 10 minutes more, divide between plates and serve.

Nutrition:

calories 240, fat 7, fiber 3, carbs 12, protein 8

Kale Eggs

Prep time: 10 minutes | **Cooking time:** 14 minutes | **Servings:** 2

Ingredients:

- 4 eggs, whisked
- ½ cup baby kale
- 2 cherry tomatoes, halved
- Salt and black pepper to the taste
- 1 tablespoon olive oil
- 2 shallots, minced
- 2 garlic cloves, minced
- 1 tablespoon chives, chopped

Directions:

1. Heat up a pan with the oil over medium heat, add the shallots and garlic and cook for 2 minutes.
2. Add the kale, eggs and the rest of the ingredients, toss, cook everything for 10 minutes more, divide between plates and serve.

Nutrition:

calories 240, fat 7, fiber 4, carbs 7, protein 12

Vanilla Bowls

Prep time: 10 minutes | **Cooking time:** 20 minutes | **Servings:** 2

Ingredients:

- ½ cup coconut, unsweetened and shredded
- 1 cup almond milk
- 1 tablespoon vanilla extract
- 2 teaspoons stevia

Directions:

1. 1. In a pan, combine the coconut with the milk and the other ingredients, stir, cook over medium heat for 20 minutes, divide into bowls and serve.

Nutrition:

calories 245, fat 12, fiber 12, carbs 2, protein 9

Chia Pudding

Prep time: 10 minutes | **Cooking time:** 20 minutes | **Servings:** 2

Ingredients:

- 2 cups almond milk
- ½ cup blackberries
- 1/3 cup chia seeds
- 1 tablespoon stevia
- 1 tablespoon vanilla extract

Directions:

1. 1. Heat up a small pot milk over medium heat, add the chia, berries and the other ingredients, toss, cook over medium heat for 20 minutes, divide into bowls and serve.

Nutrition:

calories 100, fat 0.4, fiber 4, carbs 3, protein 3

Rosemary Porridge

Prep time: 5 minutes | **Cooking time:** 20 minutes | **Servings:** 2

Ingredients:

- 1 tablespoon olive oil
- 1 cup coconut cream
- 2 scallions, chopped
- ½ cup mushrooms, halved
- ½ cup coconut, unsweetened and shredded
- A pinch of salt and black pepper
- ½ teaspoon rosemary, dried

Directions:

1. Heat up a pan with the oil over medium heat, add the scallions and mushrooms and cook for 5 minutes stirring often.
2. Add the cream and the rest of the ingredients, toss, cook over medium heat for 15 minutes more, divide into bowls and serve for breakfast.

Nutrition:

calories 230, fat 12, fiber 7, carbs 3, protein 43

Stevia and Nuts Bowls

Prep time: 5 minutes | **Cooking time:** 10 minutes | **Servings:** 2

Ingredients:

- ½ cup coconut, unsweetened and shredded
- 2 teaspoons ghee, melted
- 1 cup coconut cream
- 1 cup coconut milk
- 1 tablespoon stevia
- 1/3 cup macadamia nuts, chopped
- 1/3 cup walnuts, chopped

Directions:

1. Heat up a pan with the ghee over medium heat, add the nuts and coconut and cook for 5 minutes.
2. Add the cream and the other ingredients, toss, cook for 5 minutes more, divide into 2 bowls and serve.

Nutrition:

calories 140, fat 3, fiber 2, carbs 1.5, protein 7

Cinnamon Bowls

Prep time: 5 minutes | **Cooking time:** 4 minutes | **Servings:** 2

Ingredients:

- 1/3 cup chia seeds
- 2 cups almond milk
- 1 tablespoon stevia
- ½ teaspoon cinnamon, ground
- ¼ teaspoon vanilla extract

Directions:

1. 1. In a pan, combine the chia seeds with the milk and the other ingredients, toss, cook over medium-high heat for 4 minutes, divide into bowls and serve.

Nutrition:

calories 340, fat 12, fiber 10, carbs 3, protein 14

Blackberries Salad

Prep time: 3 minutes | **Servings:** 2

Ingredients:

- 1 cup blackberries
- 1 cup blueberries
- 2 cups baby kale
- 1 tablespoon lime juice
- 1 tablespoon avocado oil
- ½ cup cherry tomatoes, halved

Directions:

1. 1. In a bowl, combine the berries with the kale and the other ingredients, toss, divide into smaller bowls and serve.

Nutrition:

calories 344, fat 23, fiber 12, carbs 3, protein 4

Scallions Eggs

Prep time: 10 minutes | Cooking time: 20 minutes | Servings: 2

Ingredients:
- 1 tablespoon olive oil
- 2 scallions, chopped
- 4 eggs, whisked
- 1 teaspoon sweet paprika
- 1 tablespoon cilantro, chopped
- Salt and black pepper to the taste
- 1 tablespoon chives, chopped

Directions:
1. Heat up a pan with the oil over medium heat, add the scallions and the paprika and sauté for 5 minutes.
2. Add the eggs mixed with the other ingredients, toss, cook for 15 minutes more, divide between plates and serve.

Nutrition:
calories 194, fat 15.9, fiber 0.8, carbs 2.5, protein 11.6

Red Pepper Flakes Eggs

Prep time: 5 minutes | Cooking time: 20 minutes | Servings: 2

Ingredients:
- 2 spring onions, chopped
- 4 eggs, whisked
- A pinch of salt and black pepper
- 2 teaspoons ghee, melted
- A pinch of red pepper flakes, crushed

Directions:
1. Heat up a pan with the ghee over medium heat, add the spring onions and pepper flakes and sauté for 5 minutes.
2. Add the eggs and the other ingredients, toss, cook over medium heat for 15 minutes, divide between plates and serve.

Nutrition:
calories 169, fat 13.1, fiber 0.4, carbs 1.9, protein 11.4

White Mushroom and Cumin Eggs

Prep time: 10 minutes | Cooking time: 15 minutes | Servings: 2

Ingredients:
- 2 teaspoons olive oil
- 2 spring onions, chopped
- 1 cup white mushrooms, sliced
- ½ teaspoon cumin, ground
- 4 eggs, whisked
- A pinch of salt and black pepper
- ½ teaspoon rosemary, dried
- 1 tablespoon chives, chopped

Directions:
1. Heat up a pan with the oil medium heat, add the mushrooms and the spring onions and sauté for 5 minutes.
2. Add the eggs mixed with the other ingredients, toss, cook for 10 minutes more, divide between plates and serve.

Nutrition:
calories 182, fat 13.7, fiber 1, carbs 3.5, protein 12.6

Green Avocado Salad

Prep time: 5 minutes | Servings: 2

Ingredients:
- 2 cups baby spinach
- 1 avocado, peeled, pitted and cubed
- 2 spring onions, chopped
- 1 tablespoon chives, chopped
- 2 tomatoes, cubed
- A pinch of salt and black pepper
- 1 tablespoon lime juice
- 1 tablespoon olive oil

Directions:
1. 1. In a bowl, combine the spinach with the avocado, spring onions and the other ingredients, toss, divide between plates and serve.

Nutrition:
calories 299, fat 27, fiber 9.3, carbs 15.7, protein 4.2

Almonds and Berries Bowls

Prep time: 5 minutes | Servings: 2

Ingredients:
- ¼ cup almonds, chopped
- 1 cup blackberries
- 1 cup coconut cream
- 2 tablespoons chia seeds
- 1 tablespoon stevia

Directions:
1. 1. In a bowl, combine the berries with the almonds and the other ingredients, toss and serve.

Nutrition:
calories 200, fat 8.3, fiber 2, carbs 5, protein 4

Lime Zest Salad

Prep time: 5 minutes | Servings: 2

Ingredients:
- 2 cups cherry tomatoes, halved
- 1 cup black olives, pitted and haled
- ½ tablespoon oregano, chopped
- 1 tablespoon lime zest, grated
- A pinch of salt and black pepper
- 1 tablespoon olive oil
- 1 tablespoon lime juice

Directions:
1. 1. In a bowl, combine the tomatoes with the olives, oregano and the other ingredients, toss and serve.

Nutrition:
calories 400, fat 9.2, fiber 4, carbs 5.5, protein 13.2

Salmon and Cumin Eggs

Prep time: 5 minutes | Cooking time: 14 minutes | Servings: 2

Ingredients:
- ½ pound salmon fillets, boneless, and cubed
- 4 eggs, whisked
- A pinch of salt and black pepper
- 2 spring onions, chopped
- ½ teaspoon cumin, ground
- ½ teaspoon turmeric powder
- 1 tablespoon cilantro, chopped
- 1 tablespoon olive oil

Directions:
1. Heat up a pan with the oil over medium heat, add the spring onions and the salmon and cook for 4 minutes.
2. Add the eggs mixed with the rest of the ingredients, toss, cook for 10 minutes more, divide between plates and serve.

Nutrition:
calories 249, fat 16.8, fiber 0.6, carbs 1.4, protein 24.3

Shallot Salad

Prep time: 10 minutes | Cooking time: 12 minutes | Servings: 2

Ingredients:
- 2 cups baby kale
- ½ cup cherry tomatoes, halved
- 1 cucumber, sliced
- Juice of 1 lime
- 2 shallots, chopped
- 1 tablespoon avocado oil
- A pinch of salt and black pepper
- 2 tablespoons chives, chopped

Directions:
1. Heat up a pan with the oil over medium heat, add the shallots, stir and cook for 2 minutes.
2. Add the kale, tomatoes and the other ingredients, toss, cook everything for 10 minutes more, divide into bowls and serve.

Nutrition:
calories 140, fat 6.7, fiber 1, carbs 4.3, protein 10

Avocado Smoothie

Prep time: 5 minutes | **Servings:** 2

Ingredients:

- 1 cup almond milk
- 2 cups baby kale
- 1 avocado, peeled, pitted and chopped
- 1 tablespoon psyllium seeds
- ¼ cup almonds, chopped

Directions:

1. 1. In your blender, mix the almond milk with the kale and the other ingredients, pulse well, divide into 2 glasses and serve.

Nutrition:

calories 340, fat 30, fiber 7, carbs 7, protein 12

Ginger Smoothie

Prep time: 5 minutes | **Servings:** 2

Ingredients:

- 1 cup baby spinach
- 2 cucumbers, sliced
- 2 cups water
- 1 tablespoon ginger, grated
- 1 tablespoon swerve

Directions:

1. 1. In your blender, combine the spinach with the cucumber and the other ingredients, pulse well, divide into glasses and serve.

Nutrition:

calories 60, fat 2, fiber 3, carbs 3, protein 1

Micro Greens Bowls

Prep time: 3 minutes | **Servings:** 2

Ingredients:

- 1 cup micro greens
- 1 cup blackberries
- 1 cup baby spinach
- 1 small avocado, pitted, peeled and cubed
- ¼ teaspoon rosemary, dried
- A pinch of salt and black pepper
- 1 tablespoon lime juice
- 1 tablespoon olive oil

Directions:

1. 1. In a bowl, combine the micro greens with the berries, spinach and the other ingredients, toss and serve for breakfast.

Nutrition:

calories 100, fat 3, fiber 2, carbs 3, protein 5

Sweet Paprika Eggs Mix

Prep time: 10 minutes | **Cooking time:** 25 minutes | **Servings:** 2

Ingredients:

- 4 eggs, whisked
- ½ pound chicken breast, skinless, boneless and cubed
- 1 leek, sliced
- 1 tablespoon olive oil
- 2 scallions, chopped
- ½ teaspoon turmeric powder
- ½ teaspoon sweet paprika
- 1 tablespoon lime juice
- A pinch of salt and black pepper

Directions:

1. Heat up a pan with the oil over medium heat, add the scallions and the leek and cook for 5 minutes.
2. Add the meat and brown for 5 minutes more.
3. Add the rest of the ingredients, toss well, cook for 15 minutes, divide between plates and serve.

Nutrition:

calories 300, fat 23, fiber 3, carbs 4, protein 11

Nuts Bowls

Prep time: 5 minutes | **Cooking time:** 10 minutes | **Servings:** 2

Ingredients:

- 1 teaspoon cinnamon powder
- 1 cup coconut, unsweetened and shredded
- 2 tablespoons walnuts, chopped
- 1 tablespoon almonds, chopped
- 1 teaspoon stevia
- ¾ cup coconut cream

Directions:

1. 1. Heat up a pan with the cream over medium heat, add the coconut, walnuts and the other ingredients, toss, cook for 10 minutes, divide into bowls and serve for breakfast.

Nutrition:

calories 200, fat 12, fiber 4, carbs 8, protein 4.5

Sweet Avocado Salad

Prep time: 5 minutes | **Servings:** 4

Ingredients:

- 2 avocados, peeled, pitted and roughly cubed
- ½ cup coconut cream
- 2 teaspoons stevia
- 1 cup strawberries, halved
- 1 tablespoon lime juice

Directions:

1. 1. In a bowl, combine the avocado with the berries and the other ingredients, toss and serve for breakfast.

Nutrition:

calories 200, fat 7.5, fiber 4, carbs 5.7, protein 8

Seafood and Parsley Bowls

Prep time: 10 minutes | **Cooking time:** 12 minutes | **Servings:** 4

Ingredients:

- ½ pound cauliflower florets
- ½ pound shrimp, peeled and deveined
- 1 tablespoon olive oil
- 1 cup baby spinach
- 2 scallions, chopped
- 1 tablespoon balsamic vinegar
- 1 tablespoon parsley, chopped
- A pinch of salt and black pepper

Directions:

1. Heat up a pan with the oil over medium heat, add the scallions and the cauliflower and cook for 5 minutes.
2. Add the shrimp and the other ingredients, toss, cook everything for 7 minutes more, divide into bowls and serve for breakfast.

Nutrition:

calories 140, fat 9.3, fiber 3, carbs 4, protein 8

Coconut Eggs

Prep time: 10 minutes | **Cooking time:** 12 minutes | **Servings:** 2

Ingredients:

- 4 eggs, whisked
- 1 cup coconut milk
- 2 spring onions, chopped
- 1 tablespoon olive oil
- ½ teaspoon cumin, ground
- Salt and black pepper to the taste
- 1 tablespoon parsley, chopped

Directions:

1. Heat up a pan with the oil over medium heat, add the spring onions and the cumin and cook for 2 minutes.
2. Add the eggs mixed with the other ingredients, toss, cook the mix for 10 minutes more, divide between plates and serve.

Nutrition:

calories 200, fat 4, fiber 6, carbs 5, protein 10

Hard Boiled Eggs Bowl

Prep time: 10 minutes | **Servings:** 2

Ingredients:
- 2 eggs, hard boiled, peeled and cubed
- 1 cup cherry tomatoes, halved
- 1 cup baby arugula
- 2 spring onions, chopped
- 1 tablespoon olive oil
- A pinch of salt and black pepper
- 1 tablespoon balsamic vinegar
- 1 tablespoon chives, chopped

Directions:
1. In a bowl, combine the eggs with the tomatoes, arugula and the other ingredients, toss and serve for breakfast.

Nutrition:
calories 149, fat 11.7, fiber 1.7, carbs 5.5, protein 6.9

Garlic Shrimps Mix

Prep time: 5 minutes | **Cooking time:** 8 minutes | **Servings:** 2

Ingredients:
- ½ pound shrimp, peeled and deveined
- 1 red bell pepper, cut into strips
- 1 green bell pepper, cut into strips
- 1 tablespoon onion powder
- 1 tablespoon olive oil
- 1 garlic clove, minced
- Salt and black pepper to the taste
- ½ tablespoon chives, chopped

Directions:
1. Heat up a pan with the oil over medium heat, add onion powder and peppers and cook for 2 minutes.
2. Add the shrimp and the other ingredients, toss, cook for 6 minutes more, divide between plates and serve for breakfast.

Nutrition:
calories 235, fat 9.2, fiber 1.7, carbs 11.3, protein 27.2

Salmon Salad

Prep time: 5 minutes | **Servings:** 2

Ingredients:
- 1 cup smoked salmon, boneless and cut into strips
- ½ cup baby spinach
- 1 cup cherry tomatoes, halved
- 1 tablespoon balsamic vinegar
- 1 tablespoon olive oil
- 1 tablespoon chives, chopped
- A pinch of salt and black pepper

Directions:
1. 1. In a salad bowl, combine the salmon with the spinach, tomatoes and the remaining ingredients, toss and serve for breakfast.

Nutrition:
calories 80, fat 7.2, fiber 1.3, carbs 3.9, protein 1.1

Black Olives Salad

Prep time: 4 minutes | **Servings:** 2

Ingredients:
- 2 avocados, peeled, pitted and roughly cubed
- 1 cup cherry tomatoes, halved
- 1 cup black olives, pitted and halved
- 1 tablespoon olive oil
- 1 tablespoon shallots, minced
- 1 tablespoon lime juice
- A pinch of salt and black pepper
- 1 tablespoon dill, chopped

Directions:
1. 1. In a salad bowl, combine the avocados with the tomatoes, olives and the other ingredients, toss and serve for breakfast.

Nutrition:
calories 571, fat 53.6, fiber 16.8, carbs 26.7, protein 5.6

Cheese and Turkey Mix

Prep time: 10 minutes | **Cooking time:** 20 minutes | **Servings:** 2

Ingredients:
- ½ pound turkey breast, skinless, boneless and cubed
- 1 tablespoon olive oil
- 2 shallots, chopped
- 2 tablespoons mozzarella cheese, shredded
- ½ cup veggie stock
- ½ cup coconut cream
- 1 teaspoon rosemary, dried
- A pinch of salt and black pepper

Directions:
1. Heat up a pan with the oil over medium heat, add the shallots and the meat and cook for 5 minutes.
2. Add the rest of the ingredients except the cheese, stir and cook for 10 minutes more.
3. Sprinkle the cheese on top, cook the mix for 5 minutes more, divide between plates and serve.

Nutrition:
calories 398, fat 28.3, fiber 2.2, carbs 9.5, protein 28.8

Keto Passata

Prep time: 10 minutes | **Cooking time:** 25 minutes | **Servings:** 2

Ingredients:
- ½ pound chicken breast, skinless, boneless and cubed
- 2 scallions, chopped
- 2 garlic cloves, minced
- 1 cup chicken broth
- 1 red bell pepper, cut into strips
- 1 green bell pepper, cut into strips
- ½ cup tomato passata (unsweetened)
- 1 tablespoon olive oil
- A pinch of salt and black pepper
- 1 tablespoon cilantro, chopped

Directions:
1. Heat up a pot with the oil over medium heat, add the scallions, garlic and the meat and cook for 5 minutes.
2. Add the peppers and the other ingredients, toss, cook over medium heat for 20 minutes more, divide into bowls and serve for lunch.

Nutrition:
calories 242, fat 10.5, fiber 2.1, carbs 11.5, protein 26.1

Chives, Spinach, and Shrimps

Prep time: 5 minutes | **Cooking time:** 10 minutes | **Servings:** 2

Ingredients:
- ½ pound shrimp, peeled and deveined
- 1 tablespoon avocado oil
- 2 shallots, chopped
- 1 cup baby spinach
- Juice of 1 lime
- A pinch of salt and black pepper
- 1 teaspoon sweet paprika
- 1 teaspoon oregano, dried
- ¼ teaspoon onion powder
- ¼ teaspoon garlic powder
- 1 tablespoon chives, chopped

Directions:
3. Heat up a pan with the oil over medium heat, add shallots, paprika and the other ingredients except the shrimp and the spinach, toss and cook for 5 minutes.
4. Add the shrimp and the rest of the ingredients, toss, cook for 5 minutes more, divide the mix into bowls and serve.

Nutrition:
calories 156, fat 3.1, fiber 1.5, carbs 4.5, protein 26.7

Keto Vegetables and Beef Stew

Prep time: 10 minutes | **Cooking time:** 25 minutes | **Servings:** 2

Ingredients:

- 1 tablespoon olive oil
- ½ pound beef stew meat, ground
- 1 cup cherry tomatoes, halved
- 2 scallions, chopped
- 2 garlic cloves, minced
- ½ cup tomato passata (unsweetened)
- ½ teaspoon turmeric powder
- ½ teaspoon rosemary, dried
- ½ teaspoon cumin, ground
- A pinch of salt and black pepper
- ¼ teaspoon chili powder
- 1 tablespoon chives, chopped

Directions:

1. Heat up a pan with the oil over medium heat, add the meat, scallions and the garlic and cook for 5 minutes.
2. Add the tomatoes and the other ingredients, toss, cook over medium heat for 20 minutes more, divide into bowls and serve for lunch.

Nutrition:

calories 303, fat 14.6, fiber 2, carbs 6.7, protein 35.9

Basil and Shrimps Salad

Prep time: 10 minutes | **Cooking time:** 12 minutes | **Servings:** 2

Ingredients:

- 1 cup green beans, trimmed and halved
- ½ pound shrimp, peeled and deveined
- Juice of ½ lime
- 1 tablespoon olive oil
- 2 garlic cloves, minced
- 2 spring onions, chopped
- 1 tablespoon balsamic vinegar
- A pinch of salt and black pepper
- 1 cup baby spinach
- ½ teaspoon basil, dried
- 1 tablespoon chives, chopped

Directions:

1. Heat up a pan with the oil over medium heat, add the spring onions and the garlic and cook for 2 minutes.
2. Add the green beans and the other ingredients except the spinach and the shrimp and cook everything for 5 minutes more.
3. Add the shrimp and the spinach, toss, cook the mix for another 5 minutes, divide into bowls and serve for lunch.

Nutrition:

calories 227, fat 9.1, fiber 2.7, carbs 8.5, protein 27.8

Cilantro Pork Meatballs

Prep time: 10 minutes | **Cooking time:** 20 minutes | **Servings:** 2

Ingredients:

- 1 pound pork stew meat, ground
- 2 eggs, whisked
- 2 scallions, chopped
- 1 tablespoon rosemary, chopped
- 1 tablespoon cilantro, chopped
- 2 tablespoons coconut flour
- 1 cup tomato passata (unsweetened)
- 1 tablespoon olive oil

Directions:

1. In a bowl, combine the meat with the eggs, scallions and the other ingredients except the oil and the passata, stir well and shape medium meatballs out of this mix.
2. Heat up a pan with the oil over medium heat, add the meatballs, cook them for 5 minutes, add the passata, cook for 20 minutes more, divide between plates and serve for lunch.

Nutrition:

calories 614, fat 33.6, fiber 1.1, carbs 2.5, protein 72.3

Coconut Cream Soup

Prep time: 10 minutes | **Cooking time:** 25 minutes | **Servings:** 4

Ingredients:

- ½ pound white mushrooms, halved
- ¼ cup shallots, minced
- 2 garlic cloves, minced
- 1 tablespoon olive oil
- ½ teaspoon turmeric powder
- ½ teaspoon rosemary, dried
- 3 cups chicken broth
- ½ cup coconut cream
- A pinch of salt and black pepper
- 1 tablespoon ghee
- ½ teaspoon herbs de Provence

Directions:

1. Heat up a pot with the oil and the ghee over medium heat, add the shallots and the garlic and cook for 5 minutes.
2. Add the mushrooms and the other ingredients except the cream, stir, bring to a simmer and cook over medium heat for 20 minutes more.
3. Add the cream, transfer the soup to a blender, pulse well, divide into bowls and serve.

Nutrition:

calories 320, fat 8, fiber 4, carbs 3, protein 10

Keto Style Mix

Prep time: 5 minutes | **Cooking time:** 15 minutes | **Servings:** 2

Ingredients:

- ½ pound shrimp, peeled and deveined
- ½ cup shallots, chopped
- 1 cup zucchini, cubed
- ½ cup black olives, pitted and halved
- 1 tablespoon olive oil
- 1 tablespoon Italian seasoning
- ½ tablespoon rosemary, chopped
- ½ cup chicken broth
- A pinch of salt and black pepper
- 1 tablespoon garlic, minced

Directions:

1. Heat up a pan with the oil over medium heat, add the shallots and cook for 5 minutes.
2. Add the shrimp and the other ingredients, toss, cook for 10 minutes more, divide between plates and serve for lunch.

Nutrition:

calories 180, fat 8, fiber 1, carbs 4, protein 20

Soft Meatballs

Prep time: 5 minutes | **Cooking time:** 20 minutes | **Servings:** 2

Ingredients:

- 1 pound beef stew meat, ground
- 2 eggs, whisked
- 4 scallions, chopped
- 2 garlic cloves, minced
- 2 tablespoons coconut flour
- 1 tablespoon olive oil
- 1 cup baby spinach
- ½ cup tomato passata (unsweetened)
- A pinch of salt and black pepper

Directions:

1. In a bowl, combine the meat with the eggs, scallions and the other ingredients except the oil, spinach and passata, stir and shape medium meatballs out of this mix.
2. Heat up a pan with the oil over medium heat, add the meatballs and cook them for 3 minutes on each side.
3. Add the passata and the spinach, toss, cook for 14 minutes more, divide into bowls and serve for lunch.

Nutrition:

calories 200, fat 6, fiber 10, carbs 7, protein 10

Rosemary Broccoli with Beef

Prep time: 10 minutes | **Cooking time:** 25 minutes | **Servings:** 2

Ingredients:

- ½ pound beef stew meat, cubed
- 1 cup broccoli florets
- 1 avocado, peeled, pitted and cubed
- ½ cup beef stock
- 2 scallions, chopped
- 2 garlic cloves, minced
- 1 tablespoon olive oil
- 1 teaspoon rosemary, dried
- 1 teaspoon turmeric powder
- ½ teaspoon sweet paprika
- Salt and black pepper to the taste
- A pinch of lemon pepper
- 1 tablespoon chives, chopped

Directions:

1. Heat up a pan with the oil over medium heat, add the scallions and the garlic and cook for 5 minutes.
2. Add the beef and brown for 5 minutes.
3. Add the rest of the ingredients, toss, cook over medium heat for 15 minutes, divide between plates and serve.

Nutrition:

calories 250, fat 15, fiber 1, carbs 3, protein 10

Tender Tuna Mix

Prep time: 10 minutes | **Cooking time:** 20 minutes | **Servings:** 2

Ingredients:

- ¼ cup mixed red and green bell peppers, cubed
- 1 cup cherry tomatoes, halved
- ½ pound tuna fillets, boneless and cubed
- 4 scallions, chopped
- 1 tablespoon olive oil
- 1 tablespoon garlic, minced
- 1 cup chicken broth
- ½ teaspoon basil, dried
- ½ teaspoon oregano, dried
- 1 tablespoon chives, chopped
- A pinch of salt and black pepper

Directions:

1. Heat up a pan with the oil over medium heat, add the scallions and the peppers and cook for 5 minutes.
2. Add the tuna and the other ingredients, toss, cook for 15 minutes more, divide between plates and serve for lunch.

Nutrition:

calories 117, fat 7, fiber 1, carbs 2, protein 11

Aromatic Beef and Greens

Prep time: 10 minutes | **Cooking time:** 20 minutes | **Servings:** 2

Ingredients:

- ½ pound beef stew meat, ground
- 4 scallions, chopped
- 2 garlic cloves, minced
- 1 tablespoon olive oil
- 1 cup collard greens, torn
- 1 cup cherry tomatoes, halved
- 1 tablespoon balsamic vinegar
- ½ teaspoon rosemary, dried
- 1 teaspoon garam masala
- ½ teaspoon cumin, ground
- A pinch of salt and black pepper
- ¼ teaspoon sweet paprika
- 1 tablespoon cilantro, chopped

Directions:

1. Heat up a pan with the oil over medium heat, add the scallions and the garlic and cook for 5 minutes.
2. Add the meat and brown for 5 minutes more.
3. Add the rest of the ingredients, toss, cook for 10 minutes, divide into bowls and serve for lunch.

Nutrition:

calories 200, fat 6, fiber 3, carbs 1.5, protein 10

Keto Radish Salad

Prep time: 10 minutes | **Servings:** 2

Ingredients:

- 4 green onions, chopped
- ½ pound shrimp, peeled, deveined and cooked
- 1 cup radishes, halved
- Juice of ½ lemon
- Zest of ½ lemon, grated
- A pinch of salt and black pepper
- 1 tablespoon olive oil
- ½ tablespoon oregano, chopped
- 1 cup baby arugula

Directions:

1. 1. In a bowl, combine the shrimp with the radishes, onions and the other ingredients, toss and serve for lunch.

Nutrition:

calories 283, fat 23, fiber 5, carbs 3, protein 12

Mushrooms and Pork

Prep time: 10 minutes | **Cooking time:** 20 minutes | **Servings:** 4

Ingredients:

- 1 pound pork stew meat, ground
- 4 scallions, chopped
- 2 garlic cloves, minced
- 1 tablespoon avocado oil
- A pinch of salt and black pepper
- ½ teaspoon chili powder
- 1 green chili pepper, minced
- 1 cup baby spinach
- ½ cup tomato passata (unsweetened)
- ½ teaspoon chili powder
- 1 tablespoon cilantro, chopped
- ½ cup mushrooms, halved
- 1 teaspoon Italian seasoning
- 1 teaspoon red pepper flakes

Directions:

1. Heat up a pan with the oil over medium heat, add the garlic, scallions and the meat, stir and cook for 5 minutes.
2. Add the rest of the ingredients, toss, cook for 15 minutes more, divide into bowls and serve.

Nutrition:

calories 435, fat 23, fiber 7, carbs 10, protein 35

Turkey and Endives

Prep time: 5 minutes | **Cooking time:** 25 minutes | **Servings:** 2

Ingredients:

- 1 pound turkey breast, skinless, boneless and cubed
- 4 scallions, chopped
- 2 endives, shredded
- 1 tablespoon ghee, melted
- 1 tablespoon olive oil
- 2 tablespoons walnuts, toasted and chopped
- 1 teaspoon fennel seeds, crushed
- ½ teaspoon cumin, ground
- 2 tablespoons lemon juice
- A pinch of salt and black pepper
- ½ cup tomato passata (unsweetened)
- A pinch of cayenne pepper

Directions:

1. Heat up a pan with the oil and the ghee over medium heat, add the scallions, endives, fennel and cumin and cook for 5 minutes.
2. Add the turkey and the other ingredients, toss, cook for 20 minutes more, divide into bowls and serve for lunch.

Nutrition:

calories 200, fat 10, fiber 1, carbs 3, protein 7

Dill Fritters

Prep time: 5 minutes | **Cooking time:** 12 minutes | **Servings:** 2

Ingredients:

- ½ pound mushrooms, sliced
- Salt and black pepper to the taste
- 1 tablespoon coconut flour
- 1 egg, whisked
- 1 tablespoon dill, chopped
- 1 tablespoon chives, chopped
- 2 garlic cloves, minced
- 2 tablespoons olive oil

Directions:

1. In a bowl, combine the mushrooms with the egg, flour and the other ingredients except the oil, stir and shape medium fritters out of this mix.
2. Heat up a pan with the oil over medium heat, add the fritters, cook them for 6 minutes on each side, divide between plates and serve.

Nutrition:

calories 320, fat 13.32, fiber 5.2, carbs 10, protein 12.1

Stew Meat Bowls

Prep time: 10 minutes | **Cooking time:** 20 minutes | **Servings:** 2

Ingredients:

- 1 pound pork stew meat, cut into strips
- 1 avocado, peeled, pitted and cubed
- 3 scallions, chopped
- 1 tablespoon avocado oil
- ½ cup baby spinach
- A pinch of salt and black pepper
- Juice of ½ lime
- 2 garlic cloves, minced
- 1 tablespoon olive oil
- 2 tablespoons parsley, chopped

Directions:

1. Heat up a pan with the oil over medium heat, add the scallions, garlic and the meat and brown for 5 minutes.
2. Add the avocado and the other ingredients, toss, cook everything for 15 minutes more, divide between plates and serve for breakfast.

Nutrition:

calories 340, fat 28, fiber 5.3, carbs 6.3, protein 17.6

Cilantro and Eggs Mix

Prep time: 5 minutes | **Cooking time:** 20 minutes | **Servings:** 2

Ingredients:

- 1 leek, sliced
- 1 zucchini, cubed
- 4 eggs, whisked
- 1 tablespoon olive oil
- 2 scallions, chopped
- ½ teaspoon basil, dried
- ½ teaspoon oregano, dried
- Salt and black pepper to the taste
- ¼ teaspoon garlic powder
- 1 tablespoon cilantro, chopped

Directions:

1. Heat up a pan with the oil over medium heat, add the scallions, zucchini and the leek, stir and cook for 5 minutes.
2. Add the eggs and the other ingredients, toss, cook for 15 minutes more, divide between plates and serve.

Nutrition:

calories 340, fat 12, fiber 3.2, carbs 8, protein 23

Green Spread

Prep time: 5 minutes | **Cooking time:** 15 minutes | **Servings:** 2

Ingredients:

- ½ pound broccoli florets
- 2 scallions, chopped
- 1 cup almond milk
- 1 tablespoon olive oil
- ½ teaspoon chili powder
- 1 tablespoon lime juice
- A pinch of salt and black pepper

Directions:

1. Heat up a pan with the oil over medium heat, add the scallions and chili powder and cook for 2 minutes.
2. Add the broccoli and other ingredients, toss, cook everything for 13 minutes more, blend using an immersion blender, and serve as a morning spread.

Nutrition:

calories 250, fat 11.2, fiber 4, carbs 5.6, protein 6.20

Oregano and Tuna Casserole

Prep time: 10 minutes | **Cooking time:** 30 minutes | **Servings:** 2

Ingredients:

- ½ pound tuna, skinless, boneless and cubed
- 1 cup cheddar cheese, shredded
- 2 scallions, chopped
- 1 tablespoon avocado oil
- ½ cup cherry tomatoes, chopped
- 2 eggs, whisked
- ½ teaspoon cumin, ground
- ½ teaspoon oregano, dried
- 1 tablespoon chives, chopped
- Salt and black pepper to the taste

Directions:

1. Heat up a pan with the oil over medium heat, add the scallions, cumin, and oregano and cook for 2 minutes.
2. Add the tuna and cook for 3 minutes more.
3. Add the rest of the ingredients except the cheese, toss and cook for 5 minutes more.
4. Sprinkle the cheese on top, introduce the pan in the oven and bake at 380 degrees F for 20 minutes.
5. Cool the casserole down, divide between plates and serve.

Nutrition:

calories 135, fat 8.1, fiber 2.5, carbs 7.8, protein 9.5

Parmesan Eggs Mix

Prep time: 10 minutes | **Cooking time:** 20 minutes | **Servings:** 2

Ingredients:

- ½ pound chicken breast, skinless, boneless and cubed
- 2 shallots, chopped
- 1 tablespoon ghee, melted
- 4 eggs, whisked
- ½ cup parmesan, grated
- Salt and black pepper to the taste
- ½ teaspoon sweet paprika
- 1 tablespoon parsley, chopped

Directions:

1. Heat up a pan with the oil over medium heat, add the shallots, stir and cook for 5 minutes.
2. Add the meat and brown for 5 minutes more.
3. Add the rest of the ingredients, toss, cook the mix for 10 minutes more, divide between plates and serve.

Nutrition:

calories 273, fat 13.7, fiber 0.2, carbs 2.2, protein 4.5

Garam Masala Meal

Prep time: 10 minutes | **Cooking time:** 20 minutes | **Servings:** 2

Ingredients:
- ½ pound salmon fillets, boneless and cubed
- 1 cup black olives, pitted and halved
- 4 scallions, chopped
- 1 tablespoon avocado oil
- ½ teaspoon turmeric powder
- ½ teaspoon garam masala
- Juice of 1 lime
- 1 small avocado, pitted, peeled and cubed
- Salt and black pepper to the taste

Directions:
1. Heat up a pan with the oil over medium heat, add the scallions, turmeric and garam masala and cook for 5 minutes.
2. Add the salmon and the other ingredients, toss, cook for 15 minutes more, divide between plates and serve for lunch.

Nutrition:
calories 400, fat 23, fiber 0, carbs 2, protein 37

Green Beans with Chicken

Prep time: 10 minutes | **Cooking time:** 20 minutes | **Servings:** 2

Ingredients:
- ½ pound chicken breast, skinless, boneless and cubed
- 1 tablespoon olive oil
- 1 cup green beans, trimmed and halved
- ½ cup tomato passata
- (unsweetened)
- 1 tablespoon lime juice
- ¼ cup shallots, chopped
- 1 teaspoon garlic, minced
- A pinch of salt and black pepper

Directions:
1. Heat up a pan with the oil over medium heat, add the shallots and the garlic and cook for 5 minutes.
2. Add the chicken and the other ingredients, toss, cook for 15 minutes more, divide between plates and serve.

Nutrition:
calories 340, fat 30, fiber 5, carbs 3, protein 12

Keto Cheese Mix

Prep time: 10 minutes | **Cooking time:** 20 minutes | **Servings:** 2

Ingredients:
- 1 tablespoon olive oil
- 3 zucchinis, sliced
- ½ cup cheddar, shredded
- 1 teaspoon red pepper flakes
- 4 scallions, chopped
- 1 tablespoon garlic, minced
- A pinch of salt and black pepper
- 1 tablespoon basil, chopped

Directions:
1. Heat up a pan with the oil over medium heat, add the scallions and the garlic and cook for 5 minutes.
2. Add the zucchini and the other ingredients except the cheese, toss and cook for 10 minutes more.
3. Sprinkle the cheese on top, cook the mix for 5 minutes more, divide between plates and serve.

Nutrition:
calories 140, fat 3, fiber 1, carbs 1.3, protein 5

Salmon Stew

Prep time: 10 minutes | **Cooking time:** 15 minutes | **Servings:** 2

Ingredients:
- ½ pound salmon fillets, boneless, skinless and roughly cubed
- 1 cup chicken broth
- 1 tablespoon avocado oil, melted
- 3 scallions, chopped
- 1 cup kalamata olives, pitted and halved
- ½ cup cherry tomatoes, crushed
- A pinch of salt and black pepper
- 1 tablespoon cilantro, chopped
- 1 teaspoon lime juice

Directions:
1. Heat up a pan with the oil over medium heat, add the scallions and cook for 2 minutes.
2. Add the fish, stock and the other ingredients, toss, cook over medium heat for 13 minutes more, divide into bowls and serve for lunch.

Nutrition:
calories 254, fat 17, fiber 1.9, carbs 6.1, protein 12

Garlic Mix

Prep time: 10 minutes | **Cooking time:** 20 minutes | **Servings:** 4

Ingredients:
- ½ pound cod fillets, boneless
- 2 spring onions, chopped
- 1 cup baby kale
- 1 tablespoon olive oil
- 2 garlic cloves, minced
- 1 teaspoon chili powder
- ½ teaspoon sweet paprika
- A pinch of salt and black pepper

Directions:
1. Heat up a pan with the oil over medium heat, add the spring onions and the garlic and cook for 2 minutes.
2. Add the fish and cook it for 2 minutes on each side.
3. Add the rest of the ingredients, introduce the pan in the oven and cook at 360 degrees F for 16 minutes more.
4. Divide the mix between plates and serve for lunch.

Nutrition:
calories 160, fat 10, fiber 3, carbs 1, protein 12

Meat Casserole

Prep time: 10 minutes | **Cooking time:** 40 minutes | **Servings:** 2

Ingredients:
- 1 cup cheddar cheese, grated
- 1 cup zucchinis, cubed
- 2 eggs, whisked
- ½ pound pork stew meat, cubed
- 1 tablespoon avocado oil
- 2 scallions, chopped
- A pinch of salt and black pepper
- 3 garlic cloves, minced
- 1 tablespoon chives, chopped

Directions:
1. Heat up a pan with the oil over medium heat, add the scallions and the garlic and cook for 5 minutes.
2. Add the meat and brown for 5 minutes more.
3. Add the rest of the ingredients, toss, introduce the pan in the oven and cook at 370 degrees F for 30 minutes more, divide into bowls and serve.

Nutrition:
calories 455, fat 34, fiber 3, carbs 3, protein 33

Spiced Meat Stew

Prep time: 10 minutes | **Cooking time:** 35 minutes | **Servings:** 2

Ingredients:

- ½ pound beef stew meat, cubed
- 1 zucchini, cubed
- 2 spring onions, chopped
- 1 tablespoon olive oil
- 1 teaspoon sweet paprika
- ½ teaspoon cumin, ground
- ¼ teaspoon rosemary, dried
- ½ cup tomato passata (unsweetened)
- 2 cups beef stock
- 2 garlic cloves, minced
- 1 tablespoon cilantro, chopped
- A pinch of salt and black pepper
- A pinch of cayenne pepper

Directions:

1. Heat up a pot with the oil over medium heat, add the spring onions and the garlic and cook for 2 minutes.
2. Add the meat and brown for 3 minutes more.
3. Add the rest of the ingredients, toss, cook over medium heat for 30 minutes more, divide into bowls and serve for lunch.

Nutrition:

calories 500, fat 22, fiber 4, carbs 6, protein 56

Basil and Seafood Bowls

Prep time: 10 minutes | **Cooking time:** 20 minutes | **Servings:** 2

Ingredients:

- ½ pound shrimp, peeled and deveined
- ½ pound mushrooms, halved
- 3 scallions, chopped
- 1 tablespoon olive oil
- 1 cup baby spinach
- ½ cup cherry tomatoes, halved
- 1 tablespoon lime juice
- 1 tablespoon lime zest, grated
- ½ teaspoon basil, dried
- 1 tablespoon capers, drained
- 1 tablespoon chives, chopped
- A pinch of salt and black pepper
- ½ teaspoon paprika

Directions:

1. Heat up a pan with the oil over medium high heat, add the scallions and the mushrooms and cook for 10 minutes.
2. Add the shrimp, spinach and the other ingredients, toss, reduce heat for medium and cook the mix for 10 minutes more stirring often.
3. Divide the mix into bowls and serve for lunch.

Nutrition:

calories 100, fat 34, fiber 10, carbs 3, protein 10

Cabbage Soup

Prep time: 10 minutes | **Cooking time:** 25 minutes | **Servings:** 2

Ingredients:

- 1 green cabbage head, shredded
- 2 scallions, chopped
- 3 cups veggie stock
- 1 cup cherry tomatoes, halved
- ½ teaspoon sweet paprika
- 1 tablespoon olive oil
- 1 tablespoon cilantro, chopped
- A pinch of salt and black pepper

Directions:

1. Heat up a pot with the oil over medium heat, add the scallions and cook for 5 minutes.
2. Add the cabbage and the other ingredients, toss, cook the soup for 20 minutes more, divide into bowls and serve right away.

Nutrition:

calories 230, fat 34, fiber 3, carbs 5, protein 7

Kale and Garlic Soup

Prep time: 5 minutes | **Cooking time:** 15 minutes | **Servings:** 2

Ingredients:

- ½ pound shrimp, peeled and deveined
- 2 scallions, chopped
- 1 tablespoon olive oil
- 1 cup kale, torn
- 4 cherry tomatoes, halved
- 3 cups chicken broth
- Salt and black pepper to the taste
- 2 garlic cloves, minced
- 2 teaspoons thyme, dried
- 1 tablespoon cilantro, chopped

Directions:

1. Heat up a pot with the oil over medium heat, add the scallions and the garlic and cook for 3 minutes.
2. Add the kale and cook for 2 minutes more.
3. Add the shrimp and the other ingredients, toss, bring to a simmer, cook for 10 minutes, divide into bowls and serve right away.

Nutrition:

calories 270, fat 12, fiber 3, carbs 5, protein 3

Poultry and Fish Soup

Prep time: 10 minutes | **Cooking time:** 20 minutes | **Servings:** 2

Ingredients:

- 3 scallions, chopped
- 1 tablespoon olive oil
- ½ pound salmon fillets, boneless and cubed
- 4 cups chicken broth
- 1 cup cherry tomatoes, halved
- A pinch of salt and black pepper
- ½ teaspoon ginger, minced
- ½ teaspoon oregano, dried
- 1 tablespoon dill, chopped

Directions:

1. Heat up a pot with the oil over medium heat, add the scallions and the ginger and sauté for 5 minutes.
2. Add the salmon and the other ingredients, toss, bring to a simmer and cook over medium heat for 15 minutes more.
3. Divide into bowls and serve.

Nutrition:

calories 140, fat 6, fiber 1, carbs 4, protein 14

Meat and Spinach Bowls

Prep time: 10 minutes | **Cooking time:** 20 minutes | **Servings:** 2

Ingredients:

- 2 shallots, chopped
- 1 tablespoon avocado oil
- ½ pound beef stew meat, ground
- 1 green bell pepper, chopped
- 2 eggs, whisked
- 1 cup baby spinach
- ½ cup cherry tomatoes, halved
- Salt and black pepper to the taste
- 1 tablespoon chives, chopped

Directions:

1. Heat up a pan with the oil over medium heat, add the shallots and the pepper and cook for 5 minutes.
2. Add the meat and brown for 5 minutes more.
3. Add the remaining ingredients, toss, cook for 10 minutes more, divide into bowls and serve.

Nutrition:

calories 314, fat 12.6, fiber 2, carbs 7.6, protein 41.5

Jalapeno Chicken Thighs

Prep time: 10 minutes | **Cooking time:** 25 minutes | **Servings:** 2

Ingredients:

- ½ pound chicken thighs, boneless, skinless
- 1 tablespoon balsamic vinegar
- 2 spring onions, chopped
- 2 jalapenos, chopped
- 1 tablespoon olive oil
- A pinch of salt and black pepper
- 1 tablespoon lime juice
- 2 tablespoons cilantro, chopped

Directions:

1. Heat up a pan with the oil over medium heat, add the spring onions and the jalapenos, stir and cook for 5 minutes.
2. Add the meat and brown for 5 minutes more.
3. Add the rest of the ingredients, toss, cook everything for 15 minutes more, divide between plates and serve.

Nutrition:

calories 240, fat 12, fiber 5, carbs 5, protein 20

Walnuts and Beef Bowl

Prep time: 10 minutes | **Cooking time:** 25 minutes | **Servings:** 2

Ingredients:

- ½ pound beef, ground
- 1 cup green beans, trimmed and halved
- 2 spring onions, chopped
- 1 tablespoon olive oil
- ¼ cup tomato passata (unsweetened)
- 2 garlic cloves, minced
- 1 tablespoon walnuts, chopped
- Salt and black pepper to the taste
- 1 tablespoon cilantro, chopped

Directions:

1. Heat up a pan with the oil over medium heat, add the spring onions and the garlic and cook for 5 minutes.
2. Add the beef and cook for 5 minutes more.
3. Add the rest of the ingredients, toss, cook the mix for 15 minutes more, divide between plates and serve.

Nutrition:

calories 350, fat 23, fiber 6, carbs 3, protein 10

Baby Spinach and Avocado Salad

Prep time: 10 minutes | **Cooking time:** 14 minutes | **Servings:** 2

Ingredients:

- 1 tablespoon coconut oil, melted
- ½ pound white mushrooms, halved
- 1 avocado, peeled, pitted and cubed
- 1 cup cherry tomatoes, halved
- 1 cup baby spinach
- Juice of 1 lime
- 2 scallions, chopped
- 1 tablespoon balsamic vinegar
- A pinch of salt and black pepper
- 2 garlic cloves, minced

Directions:

1. Heat up a pan with the oil over medium heat, add the scallions, mushrooms and the garlic and sauté for 4 minutes.
2. Add the avocado and the other ingredients, toss, cook over medium heat for 10 minutes more, divide into bowls and serve.

Nutrition:

calories 140, fat 9, fiber 2, carbs 3, protein 4

Almond Pancakes

Prep time: 10 minutes | **Cooking time:** 10 minutes | **Servings:** 2

Ingredients:

- 2 eggs, whisked
- ½ cup strawberries, chopped
- ½ cup coconut flour
- 1 cup almond milk
- ½ teaspoon baking powder
- 1 teaspoon almond extract
- 2 teaspoons coconut oil, melted

Directions:

1. In a bowl, combine the eggs with the strawberries, flour and the other ingredients except the oil, and whisk well.
2. Heat up a pan with the oil over medium heat, add ¼ of the batter, spread into the pan, cook for 3 minutes on each side and transfer to a plate.
3. Repeat the action with the rest of the batter and serve the pancakes for breakfast.

Nutrition:

calories 266, fat 13, fiber 8, carbs 10, protein 11

Turmeric Pancakes

Prep time: 10 minutes | **Cooking time:** 10 minutes | **Servings:** 2

Ingredients:

- 1 cup zucchinis, grated
- ½ cup coconut flour
- ½ teaspoon baking powder
- 1 cup almond milk
- 1 cup coconut cream
- ½ teaspoon turmeric powder
- 2 eggs, whisked
- 2 teaspoons avocado oil
- A pinch of salt and black pepper

Directions:

1. In a bowl, combine the zucchini is with the flour, milk and the other ingredients except the oil and stir well.
2. Heat up a pan with the oil over medium heat, add ¼ of the batter, spread into the pan, cook for 3 minutes on each side, and transfer to a plate.
3. Repeat with the rest of the batter and serve the pancakes for breakfast.

Nutrition:

calories 400, fat 23, fiber 4, carbs 5, protein 3

Garlic Zucchini

Prep time: 10 minutes | **Cooking time:** 20 minutes | **Servings:** 2

Ingredients:

- 4 scallions, minced
- 1 tablespoon olive oil
- 1 garlic clove, minced
- 3 zucchinis, roughly cubed
- 1 teaspoon cumin, ground
- Salt and black pepper to the taste
- 3 cups chicken broth
- ½ cup coconut cream
- 1 tablespoon dill, chopped

Directions:

1. Heat up a pot with the oil over medium heat, add the scallions and the garlic and cook for 5 minutes.
2. Add the zucchinis and the other ingredients except the cream, stir, bring to a simmer and cook over medium heat for 15 minutes.
3. Add the cream, transfer the mix to a blender, pulse well, divide into bowls and serve.

Nutrition:

calories 140, fat 12, fiber 3, carbs 6, protein 2

Onion Powder Eggs

Prep time: 5 minutes | **Cooking time:** 16 minutes | **Servings:** 2

Ingredients:
- 2 teaspoons avocado oil
- ½ pound turkey meat, ground
- 1 teaspoon cumin, ground
- 1 teaspoon onion powder
- 2 scallions, chopped
- 2 teaspoons parsley, chopped
- 4 eggs, whisked
- A pinch of salt and black pepper

Directions:
1. Heat up a pan with the oil over medium heat, add the scallions, cumin and onion powder and cook for 5 minutes.
2. Add the meat and brown it for 5 minutes more.
3. Add the eggs and the remaining ingredients, toss, cook for 6 minutes more, divide between plates and serve.

Nutrition:
calories 280, fat 12, fiber 4, carbs 7, protein 14

Hot Eggs

Prep time: 5 minutes | **Cooking time:** 20 minutes | **Servings:** 2

Ingredients:
- 2 teaspoons avocado oil
- 1 red chili pepper, minced
- A pinch of red pepper flakes, crushed
- 2 shallots, chopped
- 4 eggs, whisked
- 1 teaspoon oregano, dried
- 1 tablespoon chives, chopped
- Salt and black pepper to the taste

Directions:
1. Heat up a pan with the oil over medium heat, add the shallots, chili pepper and pepper flakes, stir and cook for 5 minutes.
2. Add the eggs and the rest of the ingredients, toss, cook for 15 minutes more, divide between plates and serve.

Nutrition:
calories 136, fat 9.5, fiber 0.7, carbs 1.7, protein 11.3

Cheddar Cheese Bake

Prep time: 10 minutes | **Cooking time:** 30 minutes | **Servings:** 2

Ingredients:
- 2 teaspoons avocado oil
- 1 red onion, chopped
- 2 zucchinis, roughly cubed
- ½ teaspoon turmeric powder
- ½ teaspoon sweet paprika
- 4 eggs, whisked
- 1 cup cheddar cheese, shredded
- Salt and black pepper to the taste
- 2 tablespoons chives, chopped

Directions:
1. Heat up a pan with the oil over medium heat, add the onion and cook for 5 minutes.
2. Add the zucchinis and the other ingredients except the cheddar, toss and cook for 5 minutes more.
3. Sprinkle the cheese on top, introduce the pan in the oven, cook at 370 degrees F for 30 minutes, slice and serve.

Nutrition:
calories 560, fat 32, fiber 1, carbs 6, protein 20

Spinach Bowl

Prep time: 5 minutes | **Servings:** 2

Ingredients:
- 2 cups baby spinach
- 1 cup cherry tomatoes, halved
- 1 tablespoon olive oil
- 1 tablespoon lime juice
- ¼ cup raspberries
- 2 tablespoons walnuts, chopped

Directions:
1. 1. In a bowl, combine the spinach with the tomatoes and the other ingredients, toss and serve for breakfast.

Nutrition:
calories 250, fat 34, fiber 4, carbs 4, protein 5

Green Lime Omelet

Prep time: 10 minutes | **Cooking time:** 10 minutes | **Servings:** 2

Ingredients:
- 4 eggs, whisked
- 2 tablespoons basil pesto
- 2 scallions, chopped
- 1 tablespoon ghee, melted
- A pinch of salt and black pepper
- 1 tablespoon lime juice
- ½ teaspoon turmeric powder

Directions:
1. Heat up a pan with the ghee over medium high heat, add the scallions and cook for 2 minutes.
2. Add the eggs mixed with the pesto and the other ingredients, whisk, spread into the pan, cook for 4 minutes on each side, divide between plates and serve.

Nutrition:
calories 500, fat 43, fiber 6, carbs 3, protein 10

Capers and Tuna Salad

Prep time: 10 minutes | **Servings:** 4

Ingredients:
- 1 cup baby kale
- 1 avocado, peeled, pitted and cubed
- 6 ounces tuna in olive oil, drained and flaked
- 4 spring onions, chopped
- Salt and black pepper to the taste
- A pinch of chili flakes
- 1 tablespoon capers, drained
- 1 tablespoon chives, chopped

Directions:
1. 1. In a salad bowl, mix the kale with avocado, tuna and the other ingredients, toss and serve.

Nutrition:
calories 160, fat 2, fiber 1, carbs 2, protein 6

Poultry and Cucumber Salad

Prep time: 10 minutes | **Servings:** 2

Ingredients:
- ½ cup baby spinach
- ½ cup cherry tomatoes, halved
- 2 ounces rotisserie chicken, skinless, boneless and roughly chopped
- 2 tablespoons avocado oil
- 1 tablespoon lime juice
- 1 cucumber, sliced
- Salt and black pepper to the taste

Directions:
1. 1. In a bowl, combine the chicken with the spinach, tomatoes and the other ingredients, toss and serve for breakfast.

Nutrition:
calories 180, fat 12, fiber 4, carbs 5, protein 7

Turmeric Sprouts Soup

Prep time: 10 minutes | **Cooking time:** 20 minutes | **Servings:** 2

Ingredients:

- ½ pound green beans, trimmed and halved
- ½ pound Brussels sprouts, trimmed and halved
- 2 tablespoons ghee, melted
- 3 scallions, chopped
- 3 cups veggie stock
- A pinch of salt and black pepper
- 1 teaspoon oregano, dried
- ½ teaspoon turmeric powder
- 1 tablespoon chives, chopped

Directions:

1. Heat up a pot with the ghee over medium heat, add the scallions and cook for 5 minutes.
2. Add the green beans and the other ingredients, toss, bring to a simmer and cook over medium heat for 15 minutes more.
3. Divide the soup into bowls and serve.

Nutrition:

calories 400, fat 34, fiber 7, carbs 10, protein 12

Spiralized Salad

Prep time: 5 minutes | **Cooking time:** 12 minutes | **Servings:** 2

Ingredients:

- ½ pound zucchinis, cut with a spiralizer
- ½ cup cherry tomatoes, halved
- ½ cup white mushrooms, halved
- 1 tablespoon olive oil
- Juice of 1 lime
- 2 shallots, chopped
- Salt and black pepper to the taste
- 1 tablespoon basil, chopped

Directions:

1. Heat up a pan with the oil over medium high heat, add the mushrooms, shallots and tomatoes and cook for 5 minutes.
2. Add the zucchini noodles and the rest of the ingredients, toss, cook for 7 minutes more, divide into bowls and serve for breakfast.

Nutrition:

calories 90, fat 7.4, fiber 2, carbs 6.2, protein 2.4

Spiced Chicken Pan

Prep time: 5 minutes | **Cooking time:** 20 minutes | **Servings:** 2

Ingredients:

- 1 tablespoon olive oil
- ½ pound chicken breast, skinless, boneless and cubed
- 1 cup zucchinis, sliced
- 2 shallots, chopped
- 1 red chili pepper, minced
- ½ teaspoon rosemary, dried
- ½ teaspoon cumin, ground
- ½ teaspoon turmeric powder
- A pinch of salt and black pepper
- 1 tablespoon basil, chopped

Directions:

1. Heat up a pan with the oil over medium heat, add the shallots, chili pepper and the chicken and cook for 5 minutes.
2. Add the zucchinis and the other ingredients, toss, cook over medium heat for 15 minutes more, divide into bowls and serve for lunch.

Nutrition:

calories 176, fat 5.5, fiber 0.4, carbs 4.2, protein 26.5

Cream and Cauliflower Soup

Prep time: 10 minutes | **Cooking time:** 20 minutes | **Servings:** 2

Ingredients:

- 2 cups vegetable stock
- ½ pound cauliflower florets
- 2 scallions, chopped
- 1 tablespoon avocado oil
- ½ cup coconut cream
- 1 tablespoon dill, chopped
- A pinch of salt and black pepper
- Juice of 1 lime

Directions:

1. Heat up a pot with the oil over medium heat, add the scallions and cook for 2 minutes.
2. Add the cauliflower, stock and the other ingredients except the cream, stir and cook over medium heat for 18 minutes more.
3. Add the cream, blend the mix using the immersion blender, divide into bowls and serve for lunch.

Nutrition:

calories 450, fat 34, fiber 4, carbs 8, protein 12

Chicken Pan

Prep time: 5 minutes | **Cooking time:** 25 minutes | **Servings:** 2

Ingredients:

- ½ pound chicken breast, skinless, boneless and cubed
- 2 spring onions, chopped
- 1 tablespoon olive oil
- 1 cup cherry tomatoes, halved
- 1 tablespoon capers, drained
- ½ teaspoon turmeric powder
- ½ teaspoon chili powder
- 1 tablespoon cilantro, chopped
- A pinch of salt and black pepper

Directions:

1. Heat up a pan with the oil over medium heat, add the spring onions, the meat, turmeric and chili powder, toss and cook for 10 minutes.
2. Add the rest of the ingredients, toss, cook for 15 minutes more, divide between plates and serve for lunch.

Nutrition:

calories 216, fat 10.3, fiber 2, carbs 5.6, protein 25.3

Chicken Sauce

Prep time: 10 minutes | **Cooking time:** 20 minutes | **Servings:** 2

Ingredients:

- 2 shallots, chopped
- 1 tablespoon olive oil
- ½ pound chicken breast, skinless, boneless and cubed
- 3 garlic cloves, minced
- 1 cup chicken broth
- 1 tablespoon lime juice
- 1 tablespoon lime zest, grated
- 1 tablespoon cilantro, chopped

Directions:

1. Heat up a pan with the oil over medium heat, add the shallots and the garlic and cook for 5 minutes.
2. Add the meat and cook for 5 minutes more.
3. Add the rest of the ingredients, toss, cook over medium heat for 10 minutes, divide between plates and serve.

Nutrition:

calories 340, fat 12.6, fiber 6.4, carbs 7, protein 12.5

Breakfast Recipes

Crab Mix

Prep time: 10 minutes | **Servings:** 2

Ingredients:
- 2 cups crab meat, shredded
- 1 cup baby spinach
- ½ cup cherry tomatoes, halved
- ½ cup black olives, pitted and halved
- 1 tablespoon olive oil
- 1 tablespoon chives, chopped
- Juice of 1 lime
- A pinch of salt and black pepper

Directions:
1. 1. In a bowl, combine the crab meat with the spinach and the other ingredients, toss and serve for lunch.

Nutrition:
calories 200, fat 12, fiber 7, carbs 6, protein 12

Salmon and Capers Salad

Prep time: 10 minutes | **Servings:** 2

Ingredients:
- 1 cup smoked salmon, boneless and cubed
- 1 cup baby arugula
- 1 tablespoon capers, drained
- 1 cucumber, sliced
- 1 tablespoon olive oil
- 1 teaspoon balsamic vinegar
- Salt and black pepper to the taste

Directions:
1. 1. In a bowl, combine the salmon with the arugula and the other ingredients, toss and serve for lunch.

Nutrition:
calories 450, fat 43, fiber 5, carbs 4, protein 21

Vinegar Shrimps

Prep time: 5 minutes | **Cooking time:** 10 minutes | **Servings:** 2

Ingredients:
- ½ pound shrimp, peeled and deveined
- ¼ pound cherry tomatoes, halved
- 4 scallions, chopped
- 1 tablespoon olive oil
- 2 garlic cloves, minced
- ½ teaspoon turmeric powder
- ½ teaspoon oregano, dried
- 1 tablespoon balsamic vinegar
- 1 tablespoon chives, chopped

Directions:
1. Heat up a pan with the oil over medium heat, add the scallions and the garlic and cook for 2 minutes.
2. Add the shrimp and the other ingredients, toss, cook for 8 minutes, divide between plates and serve.

Nutrition:
calories 150, fat 12, fiber 5, carbs 6, protein 9

Lunch Shrimps

Prep time: 5 minutes | **Servings:** 2

Ingredients:
- 1 cup baby spinach
- ½ pound shrimp, peeled, deveined and cooked
- ½ cup cucumber, sliced
- Juice of 1 lime
- 1 tablespoon olive oil
- A pinch of salt and black pepper

Directions:
1. 1. In a salad bowl, combine the shrimp with the spinach and the other ingredients, toss and serve for lunch.

Nutrition:
calories 200, fat 14, fiber 4, carbs 2, protein 10

Cherry Tomatoes and Shrimps Bowl

Prep time: 5 minutes | **Cooking time:** 8 minutes | **Servings:** 2

Ingredients:
- 1 cup baby spinach
- 1 avocado, peeled, pitted and cubed
- ½ pound shrimp, peeled, deveined
- 2 spring onions, chopped
- 4 cherry tomatoes, halved
- 1 tablespoon avocado oil
- 1 tablespoon balsamic vinegar
- A pinch of salt and black pepper

Directions:
1. Heat up a pan with the oil over medium heat, add the spring onions and cook them for 2 minutes.
2. Add the shrimp, toss and cook for 4 minutes more.
3. Add the rest of the ingredients, toss, cook for 2 minutes, divide into bowls and serve for lunch.

Nutrition:
calories 141, fat 11.1, fiber 5.1, carbs 9.5, protein 3.6

Turmeric Eggs with Shrimps

Prep time: 10 minutes | **Cooking time:** 12 minutes | **Servings:** 2

Ingredients:
- 1 cup shrimp, peeled and deveined
- 4 eggs, whisked
- ½ teaspoon turmeric powder
- 2 spring onions, chopped
- 1 tablespoon olive oil
- Salt and black pepper to the taste
- ½ tablespoon cilantro, chopped

Directions:
1. Heat up a pan with the oil over medium heat, add the spring onions and turmeric and cook for 2 minutes.
2. Add the shrimp and cook for 3 minutes more.
3. Add the eggs and the rest of the ingredients, toss, cook for 7 minutes more, divide between plates and serve.

Nutrition:
calories 193, fat 15.8, fiber 0.7, carbs 2.2, protein 11.4

Chives Muffins

Prep time: 10 minutes | **Cooking time:** 25 minutes | **Servings:** 2

Ingredients:
- 1 tablespoon olive oil
- 1 egg
- 1 tablespoons oregano, chopped
- ½ cup almond flour
- ¼ teaspoon baking powder
- Salt and black pepper to the taste
- ½ cup coconut milk
- 1 tablespoon chives, chopped

1 tablespoon cheddar, grated

Directions:
1. In a bowl, combine the egg with the oregano, flour and the other ingredients, stir well, divide into a muffing tray, introduce in the oven at 350 degrees F for 25 minutes.
2. Leave your muffins to cool down for a few minutes, divide them between plates and serve.

Nutrition:
calories 160, fat 3, fiber 2, carbs 6, protein 10

Ghee Eggs Mix

Prep time: 5 minutes | **Cooking time:** 12 minutes | **Servings:** 2

Ingredients:
- 2 spring onions, chopped
- 4 eggs, whisked
- 1 tablespoon lemon juice
- Salt and black pepper to the taste
- 1 tablespoon ghee, melted
- 2 teaspoons lemon thyme, chopped

Directions:
1. Heat up a pan with the ghee over medium heat, add the spring onion and lemon thyme and cook for 2 minutes.
2. Add the eggs and the rest of the ingredients, toss, cook for 10 minutes more, divide between plates and serve.

Nutrition:
calories 213, fat 7, fiber 2, carbs 9, protein 8

Lime Juice and Poultry Salad

Prep time: 10 minutes | **Cooking time:** 20 minutes | **Servings:** 2

Ingredients:
- ½ pound turkey breast, skinless, boneless and cubed
- 1 cup baby spinach
- 1 tablespoon olive oil
- 1 tablespoon lime juice
- 1 avocado, peeled, pitted and cubed
- A pinch of salt and black pepper

Directions:
1. Heat up a pan over medium heat, add the turkey and cook for 5 minutes.
2. Add the rest of the ingredients, toss, cook for 15 minutes more, divide into bowls and serve for breakfast.

Nutrition:
calories 135, fat 7, fiber 2, carbs 4, protein 10

Almond and Coconut Porridge Bowls

Prep time: 5 minutes | **Cooking time:** 6 minutes | **Servings:** 2

Ingredients:
- 2 avocados, peeled, pitted and roughly mashed
- 1 cup coconut, unsweetened and shredded
- 1 cup coconut cream
- 1 cup almond milk
- ½ teaspoon vanilla extract
- 2 teaspoons stevia

Directions:
1. 1. Heat up a pan with the milk over medium heat, add the avocado, coconut and the other ingredients, whisk, cook for 6 minutes, divide into bowls and serve.

Nutrition:
calories 200, fat 12, fiber 1, carbs 1, protein 7

Sweet Omelet

Prep time: 10 minutes | **Cooking time:** 20 minutes | **Servings:** 2

Ingredients:
- 4 eggs, whisked
- 1 teaspoon sweet paprika
- A pinch of salt and black pepper
- 1 tablespoon ghee, melted
- 2 spring onions, chopped
- 1 tablespoon chives, chopped

Directions:
1. Heat up a pan with the ghee over medium heat, add the spring onions and paprika and cook for 5 minutes.
2. Add the eggs and the other ingredients, toss, spread the mix into the pan, cook for 15 minutes more, divide between plates and serve.

Nutrition:
calories 345, fat 12, fiber 1.5, carbs 8, protein 13.3

Turmeric Brussels Sprouts

Prep time: 10 minutes | **Cooking time:** 20 minutes | **Servings:** 2

Ingredients:
- ½ pound Brussels sprouts, trimmed and halved
- 2 garlic cloves, minced
- 2 tablespoons ghee, melted
- 1 cup chicken broth
- 1 tablespoon balsamic vinegar
- Salt and black pepper to the taste
- ½ teaspoon cumin, ground
- ½ teaspoon rosemary, dried
- 1 teaspoon turmeric powder
- 1 tablespoon cilantro, chopped

Directions:
1. 1. Heat up a pan with the ghee over medium heat, add the garlic, sprouts and the other ingredients, toss, cook for 20 minutes, divide between plates and serve.

Nutrition:
calories 300, fat 20, fiber 6, carbs 5, protein 10

Basil Salad

Prep time: 5 minutes | **Servings:** 2

Ingredients:
- 1 cup cherry tomatoes, halved
- 1 tablespoon chives, chopped
- A pinch of salt and black pepper
- ½ teaspoon basil, dried
- 1 avocado, peeled, pitted and roughly cubed
- A pinch of salt and black pepper
- 2 spring onions, chopped
- 1 tablespoon avocado oil

Directions:
1. 1. In a bowl, combine the tomatoes with the chives and the other ingredients, toss and serve for breakfast.

Nutrition:
calories 236, fat 20.7, fiber 8.6, carbs 13.8, protein 3.1

Baby Spinach and Chicken Bowls

Prep time: 10 minutes | **Servings:** 2

Ingredients:
- 2 ounces rotisserie chicken, skinless, boneless and shredded
- 1 tablespoon olive oil
- 1 tablespoon lime juice
- 1 cup baby spinach
- 1 cup cherry tomatoes, halved
- 1 cucumber, sliced
- 1 small avocado, pitted, peeled and cubed
- Salt and black pepper to the taste

Directions:
1. 1. In a bowl, combine the chicken with the oil, lime juice and the other ingredients, toss and serve for breakfast.

Nutrition:
calories 200, fat 32, fiber 6, carbs 4, protein 5

Baby Spinach Soup

Prep time: 10 minutes | **Servings:** 2

Ingredients:
- 2 avocados, peeled, pitted and mashed
- 1 cucumber, chopped
- 1 cup baby spinach
- 2 cups veggie stock, warm
- ½ cup coconut cream
- 1 tablespoon chives, chopped
- A pinch of salt and black pepper
- A pinch of garlic powder
- ½ teaspoon sweet paprika

Directions:
1. 1. In a blender, combine the avocados with the cucumber and the other ingredients, pulse well, divide into bowls and serve for lunch.

Nutrition:
calories 200, fat 37, fiber 12, carbs 4, protein 10

Chili Powder Meat

Prep time: 5 minutes | **Cooking time:** 20 minutes | **Servings:** 2

Ingredients:

- ½ pound beef stew meat, cubed
- 1 tablespoon olive oil
- 1 red chili pepper, minced
- ½ teaspoon chili powder
- 1 cup cherry tomatoes, halved
- 1 handful cilantro, chopped
- 1 garlic clove, minced
- 1 tablespoon cilantro, chopped
- A pinch of salt and black pepper

Directions:

1. Heat up a pan with the oil over medium heat, add the meat and brown for 5 minutes.
2. Add the chili pepper and the other ingredients, toss, cook over medium heat for 15 minutes more, divide between plates and serve.

Nutrition:

calories 200, fat 5, fiber 6, carbs 5, protein 3

Poultry Stew

Prep time: 10 minutes | **Cooking time:** 30 minutes | **Servings:** 2

Ingredients:

- ½ pound turkey breast, skinless, boneless and cubed
- 1 cup broccoli florets
- 3 scallions, chopped
- 1 tablespoon olive oil
- 2 garlic cloves, minced
- 1 cup chicken broth
- ¼ cup tomato passata (unsweetened)
- 1 tablespoon cilantro, chopped
- ¼ teaspoon cumin, ground
- A pinch of salt and black pepper

Directions:

1. Heat up a pan with the oil over medium heat, add the scallions, garlic and the meat and cook for 5 minutes.
2. Add the stock and the other ingredients, toss, cook over medium heat for 25 minutes, divide into bowls and serve.

Nutrition:

calories 270, fat 43, fiber 5, carbs 4, protein 6

Turkey Stew

Prep time: 10 minutes | **Cooking time:** 20 minutes | **Servings:** 2

Ingredients:

- ½ pound turkey breast, skinless, boneless and cubed
- 1 tablespoon olive oil
- 2 scallions, chopped
- 1 tablespoon lime juice
- 1 tablespoon dill, chopped
- ½ cup chicken broth
- ½ cup tomato passata (unsweetened)
- 1 cup baby spinach
- A pinch of salt and black pepper

Directions:

1. Heat up a pan with the oil over medium heat, add the scallions and the meat and brown for 5 minutes.
2. Add the lime juice and the other ingredients, toss, cook over medium heat for 15 minutes more, divide into bowls and serve.

Nutrition:

calories 380, fat 40, fiber 5, carbs 1, protein 17

Aromatic Basil Shrimps

Prep time: 10 minutes | **Cooking time:** 10 minutes | **Servings:** 2

Ingredients:

- ½ pound shrimp, peeled and deveined
- 2 zucchinis, cubed
- 2 scallions, chopped
- 2 tablespoons olive oil
- Salt and black pepper to the taste
- 2 garlic cloves, minced
- Juice of ½ lemon
- ½ teaspoon sweet paprika
- 1 tablespoon basil, chopped

Directions:

1. Heat up a pan with the oil over medium heat, add the scallions and garlic and cook for 2 minutes.
2. Add the shrimp and the other ingredients, toss, cook over medium heat for 8 minutes more, divide between plates and serve.

Nutrition:

calories 300, fat 20, fiber 6, carbs 3, protein 10

Parsley Fish Stew

Prep time: 5 minutes | **Cooking time:** 20 minutes | **Servings:** 2

Ingredients:

- ½ pound cod fillets, boneless and roughly cubed
- 2 shallots, chopped
- 1 tablespoon olive oil
- 1 cup cherry tomatoes, halved
- 1 cup chicken broth
- 2 garlic cloves, minced
- 1 cup tomato passata (unsweetened)
- ½ teaspoon oregano, dried
- 1 tablespoon parsley, chopped
- A pinch of salt and black pepper

Directions:

1. Heat up a pot with the oil over medium heat, add the shallots and the garlic and sauté for 5 minutes.
2. Add the fish and the other ingredients, toss, cook over medium heat for 15 minutes more, divide into bowls and serve.

Nutrition:

calories 456, fat 32, fiber 2, carbs 6, protein 12

Curry Turkey

Prep time: 10 minutes | **Cooking time:** 25 minutes | **Servings:** 2

Ingredients:

- 1 tablespoon olive oil
- ½ pound turkey breast, skinless, boneless and cubed
- 2 scallions, chopped
- 2 garlic cloves, minced
- 1 cup chicken broth
- 2 cups coconut milk
- 1 tablespoon lime juice
- 1 tablespoon cilantro, chopped
- 1 tablespoon ginger, grated
- 2 tablespoons yellow curry paste
- 1 teaspoon turmeric powder

Directions:

1. Heat up a pot with the oil over medium high heat, add the scallions, garlic and the ginger and cook for 5 minutes.
2. Add the meat and the rest of the ingredients, toss, cook for 20 minutes more, divide into bowls and serve for lunch.

Nutrition:

calories 430, fat 22, fiber 4, carbs 7, protein 53

Parsley Soup

Prep time: 10 minutes | **Cooking time:** 30 minutes | **Servings:** 2

Ingredients:

- ½ pound beef stew meat, cubed
- 2 scallions, chopped
- 1 tablespoon olive oil
- 2 garlic cloves, minced
- 3 cups beef stock
- A pinch of salt and black pepper
- 2 tablespoons parsley, chopped
- 1 tablespoon lime juice

Directions:

1. Heat up a pot with the oil over medium heat, add the scallions, garlic and the meat and cook for 5 minutes.
2. Add the rest of the ingredients except the parsley, bring to a simmer and cook over medium heat for 20 minutes.
3. Ladle the soup into bowls, sprinkle the parsley on top and serve.

Nutrition:

calories 287, fat 14, fiber 2, carbs 7, protein 12

Passata Soup

Prep time: 5 minutes | **Cooking time:** 25 minutes | **Servings:** 4

Ingredients:

- 2 scallions, chopped
- 1 tablespoon olive oil
- ½ pound broccoli florets
- 4 cups veggie stock
- Salt and black pepper to the taste
- 2 garlic cloves, minced
- 1 cup tomato passata (unsweetened)
- ½ teaspoon sweet paprika
- 1 tablespoon cilantro, chopped

Directions:

1. Heat up a pot with the oil over medium heat, add the scallions and the garlic and cook for 5 minutes.
2. Add the broccoli and the other ingredients, stir, bring to a simmer and cook over medium heat for 20 minutes more.
3. Divide into soup bowls and serve hot.

Nutrition:

calories 350, fat 34, fiber 7, carbs 7, protein 11

White Mushrooms Stew

Prep time: 10 minutes | **Cooking time:** 25 minutes | **Servings:** 2

Ingredients:

- ½ pound white mushrooms, halved
- 3 scallions, chopped
- 2 garlic cloves, minced
- 1 cup tomato passata (unsweetened)
- 1 tablespoon lime zest, grated
- A pinch of salt and black pepper
- ½ cup vegetable stock
- 1 green bell pepper, chopped
- 1 tablespoon cilantro, chopped

Directions:

1. Heat up a pot with the scallions and the garlic and sauté for 5 minutes.
2. Add the mushrooms and cook them for 5 minutes more.
3. Add the rest of the ingredients, toss, cook over medium heat fro 15 minutes more, divide into bowls and serve for lunch.

Nutrition:

calories 155, fat 11, fiber 6, carbs 8, protein 5

Minced Garlic and Scallions Beef

Prep time: 5 minutes | **Cooking time:** 15 minutes | **Servings:** 2

Ingredients:

- 1 pound beef stew meat, cut into strips
- 1 tablespoon olive oil
- ½ cup beef stock
- 4 scallions, chopped
- 2 tablespoons mustard
- Salt and black pepper to the taste
- 2 garlic cloves, minced
- 1 teaspoon red pepper flakes
- 1 tablespoon chives, chopped

Directions:

1. Heat up a pan with the oil over medium heat, add the scallions and the garlic and cook for 2 minutes.
2. Add the meat and cook for 3 minutes more.
3. Add the rest of the ingredients, toss, cook for 10 minutes more, divide into bowls and serve for lunch.

Nutrition:

calories 435, fat 23, fiber 7, carbs 10, protein 35

Capers Mix

Prep time: 5 minutes | **Cooking time:** 15 minutes | **Servings:** 2

Ingredients:

- ½ pound tuna fillets, boneless, skinless and roughly cubed
- 2 spring onions, chopped
- 1 tablespoon olive oil
- 1 tablespoon lime juice
- 1 cup baby spinach
- A pinch of salt and black pepper
- 1 cup cherry tomatoes, halved
- 1 tablespoon capers, drained

Directions:

1. Heat up a pan with the oil over medium heat, add the spring onions and cook for 2 minutes.
2. Add the tuna and the other ingredients, toss, cook everything for 13 minutes more, divide into bowls and serve for lunch.

Nutrition:

calories 200, fat 65, fiber 4, carbs 14, protein 12

Ground Beef Bowl

Prep time: 10 minutes | **Cooking time:** 20 minutes | **Servings:** 2

Ingredients:

- ½ pound beef, ground
- 2 spring onions, chopped
- 1 tablespoon avocado oil
- 1 cup mushrooms, sliced
- Salt and black pepper to the taste
- ½ teaspoon smoked paprika
- 1 tablespoon chives, chopped
- ½ cup tomato passata (unsweetened)

Directions:

1. Heat up a pan with the oil over medium heat, add the spring onions and the beef, stir and brown for 5 minutes.
2. Add the mushrooms and the other ingredients, toss, cook over medium heat for 15 minutes, divide into bowls and serve.

Nutrition:

calories 600, fat 23, fiber 8, carbs 22, protein 43

Lime Juice and Chives Salad

Prep time: 10 minutes | **Cooking time:** 14 minutes | **Servings:** 2

Ingredients:

- 1 turkey breast, skinless, boneless, cooked and cut into strips
- 2 spring onions, chopped
- 1 tablespoon olive oil
- 1 cup cherry tomatoes, halved
- 1 cup baby kale
- 2 tablespoons lime juice
- 1 tablespoon balsamic vinegar
- 1 tablespoon chives, chopped
- Salt and black pepper to the taste

Directions:

1. Heat up a pan with the oil over medium heat, add the spring onions and the meat and cook for 4 minutes.
2. Add the kale and the other ingredients, toss, cook over medium heat for 10 minutes more, divide into bowls and serve.

Nutrition:

calories 200, fat 10, fiber 1.54, carbs 3, protein 7

Avocado and Eggs

Prep time: 10 minutes | **Cooking time:** 25 minutes | **Servings:** 2

Ingredients:

- ½ pound beef stew meat, cut into strips
- 4 eggs, whisked
- ½ teaspoon sweet paprika
- ½ teaspoon oregano, dried
- 1 small avocado, pitted, peeled and cubed
- 2 scallions, chopped
- 1 tablespoon olive oil
- 1 tablespoon chives, chopped
- Salt and black pepper to the taste

Directions:

1. Heat up a pan with oil, over medium heat, add the scallions and the meat and cook for 10 minutes.
2. Add the eggs and the other ingredients, toss, cook for 15 minutes more, stirring often, divide between plates and serve.

Nutrition:

calories 200, fat 34, fiber 10, carbs 3, protein 20

Ilspice Zucchini

Prep time: 5 minutes | **Cooking time:** 12 minutes | **Servings:** 2

Ingredients:

- 1 tablespoon olive oil
- 2 scallions, chopped
- 1 tablespoon cilantro, chopped
- 2 zucchinis, roughly cubed
- 1 teaspoon cumin, ground
- 1 teaspoon allspice, ground
- Salt and black pepper to the taste
- 1 tablespoons dill, chopped

Directions:

1. Heat up a pan with the oil over medium heat, add the scallions, cumin and allspice, stir and cook for 2 minutes.
2. Add the zucchini and the other ingredients, toss, cook everything for 10 minutes more, divide between plates and serve for breakfast.

Nutrition:

calories 140, fat 6, fiber 2, carbs 10, protein 12

Almond and Vegetables Muffins

Prep time: 10 minutes | **Cooking time:** 20 minutes | **Servings:** 2

Ingredients:

- 2 eggs, whisked
- 1 red onion, chopped
- ½ cup almond milk
- 1 zucchini, grated
- Salt and black pepper to the taste
- ½ teaspoon baking soda
- ½ cup almond flour

Directions:

1. In a bowl, combine the zucchini with the eggs and the other ingredients and stir well.
2. Divide the mix into a muffin tray, introduce in the oven at 350 degrees F and bake for 20 minutes.
3. Divide the muffins between plates and serve them for breakfast.

Nutrition:

calories 200, fat 7, fiber 4, carbs 7, protein 5

Ketogenic Lunch Recipes

Beef and Spinach Salad

Prep time: 5 minutes | **Cooking time:** 25 minutes | **Servings:** 2

Ingredients:

- ½ pound beef stew meat, cut into strips
- 1 cup baby spinach
- 1 cup cherry tomatoes, halved
- 1 tablespoon avocado oil
- 2 spring onions, chopped
- 1 cucumber, sliced
- A pinch of salt and black pepper
- 1 tablespoon balsamic vinegar

Directions:

1. Heat up a pan with the oil over medium heat, add the spring onions and the meat and cook for 10 minutes.
2. Add the rest of the ingredients, toss, cook everything for 15 minutes more, divide into bowls and serve for lunch.

Nutrition:

calories 269, fat 8.4, fiber 2.9, carbs 11.1, protein 37

Scallions and Seafood Salad

Prep time: 5 minutes | **Cooking time:** 8 minutes | **Servings:** 2

Ingredients:

- 1 tablespoon olive oil
- ½ pound shrimp, peeled and deveined
- 1 cup baby spinach
- 2 scallions, chopped
- ½ cup cherry tomatoes, halved
- 1 teaspoon sweet paprika
- Salt and black pepper to the taste
- 1 tablespoon chives, chopped

Directions:

1. Heat up a pan with the oil over medium heat, add the scallions, tomatoes and paprika, toss and sauté for 2 minutes.
2. Add the shrimp and the other ingredients, toss, cook for 6 minutes more, divide into bowls and serve.

Nutrition:

calories 215, fat 9.3, fiber 1.7, carbs 5.8, protein 27.1

Morning Waffles

Prep time: 10 minutes | **Cooking time:** 10 minutes | **Servings:** 2

Ingredients:

- 2 eggs, whisked
- 1 tablespoon almond milk
- ¼ teaspoon baking powder
- 1 cup cherry tomatoes, chopped
- 2 tablespoons coconut flour
- ½ cup ghee, melted
- A pinch of salt and black pepper

Directions:

1. In a bowl, combine the eggs with the almond milk and the other ingredients and whisk really well.
2. Pour ¼ of this in the waffle iron and cook for about 4 minutes.
3. Repeat with the rest of the batter and serve your waffles right away.

Nutrition:

calories 240, fat 23, fiber 2, carbs 4, protein 7

Paprika Chicken Thighs

Prep time: 10 minutes | **Cooking time:** 20 minutes | **Servings:** 2

Ingredients:

- ½ pound chicken thighs, boneless and skinless
- ½ cup chicken broth
- A pinch of salt and black pepper
- ½ teaspoon garlic powder
- ½ teaspoon sweet paprika
- 1 teaspoon cayenne pepper
- 1 tablespoon olive oil
- 1 tablespoon cilantro, chopped

Directions:

1. 1. Heat up a pan with the oil over medium heat, add the chicken, stock, salt and pepper and the other ingredients, toss, cook for 20 minutes, divide between plates and serve.

Nutrition:

calories 200, fat 45, fiber 12, carbs 1, protein 22

Kalamata and Chicken Salad

Prep time: 10 minutes | **Servings:** 2

Ingredients:

- 1 avocado, pitted, peeled and sliced
- ½ cup cherry tomatoes, halved
- ½ pound chicken breast, skinless, boneless, cooked and shredded
- ½ cup kalamata olives, pitted and halved
- Juice of 1 lime
- 1 tablespoon chives, chopped
- 1 tablespoon olive oil
- Salt and black pepper to the taste

Directions:

1. 1. In a salad bowl, combine the avocado with the chicken, olives and the other ingredients, toss and serve for lunch.

Nutrition:

calories 334, fat 23, fiber 4, carbs 3, protein 18

Tender Keto Muffins

Prep time: 10 minutes | **Cooking time:** 30 minutes | **Servings:** 2

Ingredients:

- 2 tablespoons ghee, melted
- 1 cup baby spinach
- 4 eggs, whisked
- Salt and black pepper to the taste
- 2 spring onions, chopped
- ½ cup almond milk
- ½ cup almond flour
- ½ teaspoon baking powder
- 1 tablespoon chives, chopped

Directions:

1. In a bowl, combine the eggs with the spinach, ghee and the other ingredients, whisk well and divide into a muffin tray.
2. Introduce in the oven and bake at 380 degrees F for 30 minutes.
3. Serve for breakfast right away.

Nutrition:

calories 440, fat 32, fiber 0, carbs 12, protein 12

Green Onions Shrimp

Prep time: 4 minutes | **Cooking time:** 8 minutes | **Servings:** 2

Ingredients:

- ½ cup green onions, chopped
- ½ pound shrimp, peeled and deveined
- 1 tablespoon basil pesto
- ½ tablespoons balsamic vinegar
- 1 tablespoon olive oil
- Salt and black pepper to the taste
- 1 tablespoon chives, chopped

Directions:

1. Heat up a pan with the oil over medium heat, add the green onions and cook them for 2 minutes.
2. Add the shrimp and the other ingredients, toss, cook over medium heat for 6 minutes more, divide into bowls and serve for lunch.

Nutrition:

calories 467, fat 38.1, fiber 8.3, carbs 14.9, protein 4.3

Chili Pepper Soup

Prep time: 10 minutes | **Cooking time:** 25 minutes | **Servings:** 2

Ingredients:

- ½ pound green beans, trimmed
- 1 tablespoon olive oil
- 2 shallots, chopped
- 1 cup cherry tomatoes, halved
- 3 cups vegetable stock
- Juice from 1 lime
- 1 red chili pepper, minced
- 1 tablespoon cilantro, chopped

Directions:

1. Heat up a pot with the oil over medium heat, add the shallots and cook for 5 minutes.
2. Add the green beans and the other ingredients, toss, cook over medium heat for 20 minutes, divide into bowls and serve.

Nutrition:

calories 300, fat 5, fiber 6, carbs 3, protein 6

Mix of Seeds Bowls

Prep time: 5 minutes | **Cooking time:** 10 minutes | **Servings:** 2

Ingredients:

- ½ cup almonds, chopped
- 2 avocados, peeled, pitted and cubed
- ½ cup pepitas
- 2 tablespoons chia seeds
- 1 cup almond milk
- 1 tablespoon lime zest, grated
- ½ cup walnuts, chopped
- ½ cup coconut, flaked and unsweetened
- ¼ cup sunflower seeds
- ½ teaspoon nutmeg

Directions:

1. 1. In a pan, combine the almonds with the avocados and the other ingredients, toss, cook over medium heat for 10 minutes, divide into bowls and serve for breakfast.

Nutrition:

calories 340, fat 32, fiber 12, carbs 20, protein 20

Bell Peppers Scrambled Eggs

Prep time: 10 minutes | **Cooking time:** 12 minutes | **Servings:** 2

Ingredients:

- 4 eggs, whisked
- 1 tablespoon olive oil
- 1 red onion, chopped
- 1 red bell pepper, chopped
- 1 green bell pepper, chopped
- 1 orange bell pepper, chopped
- Salt and black pepper to the taste
- ½ cup spinach, chopped
- 1 tablespoon chives, chopped

Directions:

1. Heat up a pan with the oil over medium heat, add the peppers and the onion and sauté for 2 minutes.
2. Add the eggs and the other ingredients, whisk well, cook for 10 minutes more, divide between plates and serve.

Nutrition:

calories 350, fat 23, fiber 1, carbs 5, protein 22

Garlic Frittata

Prep time: 10 minutes | **Cooking time:** 30 minutes | **Servings:** 2

Ingredients:

- 4 eggs, whisked
- 1 cup cheddar cheese, shredded
- ¼ cup mozzarella, shredded
- 2 spring onions, chopped
- 1 tablespoon olive oil
- 1 red onion, chopped
- 2 garlic cloves, minced
- Salt and black pepper to the taste
- 1 red chili pepper, minced
- 1 tablespoon cilantro, chopped

Directions:

1. In a bowl, combine the eggs with the cheese and the other ingredients, whisk and pour into a pan greased with the oil.
2. Spread well into the pan, cook the frittata at 375 degrees F for 30 minutes, cool down, slice and serve.

Nutrition:

calories 298, fat 2, fiber 1, carbs 6, protein 18

Cilantro Eggs

Prep time: 5 minutes | **Cooking time:** 12 minutes | **Servings:** 2

Ingredients:

- 1 tablespoon ghee, melted
- 2 scallions, chopped
- 2 spring onions, chopped
- 4 eggs, whisked
- 1 green bell pepper, chopped
- Salt and black pepper to the taste
- 1 teaspoon sweet paprika
- 1 tablespoon cilantro, chopped

Directions:

1. Heat up a pan with the ghee over medium heat, add the scallions and spring onions and cook for 2 minutes.
2. Add the eggs and the other ingredients, toss, cook for 10 minutes more, divide between plates and serve.

Nutrition:

calories 300, fat 12, fiber 3.4, carbs 22, protein 14

Shrimps and Vegetables

Prep time: 10 minutes | **Cooking time:** 10 minutes | **Servings:** 2

Ingredients:

- ½ pound shrimp, peeled and deveined
- 4 asparagus spears, trimmed and halved
- 1 tablespoon olive oil
- 1 tablespoon shallots, chopped
- ½ cup cherry tomatoes, halved
- A pinch of salt and black pepper
- A pinch of cayenne pepper

Directions:

1. Heat up a pan with the oil over medium heat, add the shallots and sauté for 2 minutes.
2. Add the shrimp and the other ingredients, toss, cook for 8 minutes more, divide between plates and serve.

Nutrition:

calories 150, fat 13, fiber 6, carbs 2, protein 3

Bell Peppers Saute

Prep time: 5 minutes | **Cooking time:** 20 minutes | **Servings:** 2

Ingredients:

- ½ pound bell peppers, cut into strips
- 1 cup vegetable stock
- 1 tablespoon olive oil
- 3 scallions, chopped
- ½ cup tomato passata
- (unsweetened)
- A pinch of salt and black pepper
- 2 garlic cloves, minced
- 1 cup cherry tomatoes, halved
- 1 tablespoon parsley, chopped

Directions:

1. Heat up a pan with the oil over medium heat, add the scallions and the garlic and cook for 5 minutes.
2. Add the peppers and the other ingredients, toss, cook for 15 minutes more, divide into bowls and serve for lunch.

Nutrition:

calories 357, fat 23, fiber 5, carbs 6.3, protein 1

Cucumbers and Olives Salad

Prep time: 5 minutes | **Cooking time:** 8 minutes | **Servings:** 2

Ingredients:

- ½ pound shrimp, peeled and deveined
- 2 cucumbers, sliced
- Juice of ½ lime
- 1 tablespoon olive oil
- 1 cup kalamata olives, pitted and halved
- 1 tablespoon chives, chopped
- A pinch of salt and black pepper

Directions:

1. Heat up a pan with the oil over medium heat, add the shrimp, cucumbers and the other ingredients, toss, cook for 8 minutes more, divide into bowls and serve.

Nutrition:

calories 230, fat 13.4, fiber 12, carbs 5, protein 6.7

Arugula Salad

Prep time: 10 minutes | **Servings:** 2

Ingredients:

- ½ pound shrimp, peeled, deveined and cooked
- 2 tablespoons walnuts, chopped
- 1 cup baby arugula
- ½ cup cherry tomatoes, halved
- 1 avocado, peeled, pitted and cubed
- 1 tablespoon olive oil
- 1 tablespoon lime juice
- A pinch of salt and black pepper

Directions:

1. In a salad bowl, combine the shrimp with the walnuts, arugula and the other ingredients, toss and serve for lunch.

Nutrition:

calories 250, fat 23, fiber 4, carbs 4, protein 5

White Mushrooms and Lamb Mix

Prep time: 10 minutes | **Cooking time:** 30 minutes | **Servings:** 2

Ingredients:

- ½ pound lamb shoulder, cubed
- 1 tablespoon olive oil
- 1 cup white mushrooms, halved
- Juice of ½ lime
- A pinch of salt and black pepper
- ½ cup veggie stock
- ½ teaspoon sweet paprika
- 1 tablespoon thyme, chopped

Directions:

1. Heat up a pan with the oil over medium heat, add the meat and brown for 5 minutes.
2. Add the mushrooms and the other ingredients, toss, cook for 25 minutes more, divide everything between plates and serve.

Nutrition:

calories 110, fat 7, fiber 4, carbs 2, protein 10

Walnuts Salad

Prep time: 10 minutes | **Servings:** 2

Ingredients:

- ½ pound shrimp, peeled, deveined and cooked
- 1 cup radishes, halved
- 1 cup cherry tomatoes, halved
- 1 cup baby spinach
- 1 tablespoon lime juice
- 1 tablespoon olive oil
- Salt and black pepper to the taste
- 2 tablespoons walnuts, toasted and chopped

Directions:

1. In a bowl, combine the shrimp with the radishes and the other ingredients, toss and serve for lunch.

Nutrition:

calories 200, fat 14, fiber 4, carbs 5, protein 6

Lemon Seabass with Avocado

Prep time: 5 minutes | **Cooking time:** 20 minutes | **Servings:** 2

Ingredients:

- 1 pound sea bass fillets, boneless and skinless
- 1 avocado, peeled, pitted and cubed
- 1 tablespoon olive oil
- ½ cup shallots, chopped
- ½ cup tomato passata (unsweetened)
- 1 tablespoon lemon juice
- A pinch of salt and black pepper
- ¼ teaspoon turmeric powder

Directions:

1. Heat up a pan with the oil over medium heat, add the shallots and cook for 5 minutes.
2. Add the sea bass and the other ingredients, toss, cook for 15 minutes more, divide into bowls and serve.

Nutrition:

calories 230, fat 34, fiber 12, carbs 5, protein 27

Ketogenic Side Dish Recipes

Basil Salad

Prep time: 10 minutes | **Servings:** 2

Ingredients:

- 2 avocados peeled, pitted and cubed
- 1 cup cherry tomatoes, halved
- 3 spring onions, chopped
- Juice of 1 lime
- 1 tablespoon basil, chopped
- 1 tablespoon olive oil
- A pinch of cayenne pepper
- A pinch of salt and black pepper

Directions:

1. 1. In a bowl, combine the avocados with the tomatoes and the other ingredients, toss, divide between plates and serve as a side salad.

Nutrition:

calories 150, fat 5.3, fiber 4, carbs 4.7, protein 7.6

Salad with Lime Juice

Prep time: 10 minutes | **Servings:** 2

Ingredients:

- 1 pound broccoli florets, steamed
- 2 garlic cloves, minced
- Juice of 1 lime
- Zest of 1 lime, grated
- 1 teaspoon chili powder
- 1 tablespoon olive oil
- A pinch of salt and black pepper
- 1 tablespoon dill, chopped

Directions:

1. In a bowl, combine the broccoli with the garlic and the other ingredients, and toss.
2. Divide the mix between plates and serve.

Nutrition:

calories 118, fat 2, fiber 3, carbs 1, protein 6

Paprika Asparagus

Prep time: 5 minutes | **Cooking time:** 10 minutes | **Servings:** 2

Ingredients:

- ½ pound asparagus spears, trimmed and halved
- 1 tablespoon avocado oil
- Juice of 1 lime
- Zest of 1 lime, grated
- ½ teaspoons sweet paprika
- 1 tablespoon chives, chopped

Directions:

1. 1. Heat up a pan with the oil over medium high heat, add the asparagus, lime juice and the other ingredients, toss, cook for 10 minutes, divide between plates and serve.

Nutrition:

calories 200, fat 4, fiber 6, carbs 2, protein 12

Spring Onions Salad

Prep time: 5 minutes | **Servings:** 2

Ingredients:

- 1 pound cherry tomatoes, halved
- 3 spring onions, chopped
- 1 tablespoon olive oil
- 1 tablespoon dill, chopped
- ½ teaspoon cayenne pepper
- A pinch of salt and black pepper
- 1 tablespoon chives, chopped

Directions:

1. 1. In a bowl, combine the tomatoes with the spring onions, oil and the other ingredients, toss and serve as a side dish.

Nutrition:

calories 72, fat 3.9, fiber 2.4, carbs 9.5, protein 1.8

Kale Saute

Prep time: 10 minutes | **Cooking time:** 20 minutes | **Servings:** 2

Ingredients:

- 1 pound kale, torn
- ¼ cup shallots, minced
- 2 garlic cloves, minced
- Juice of ½ lime
- 1 tablespoon olive oil
- ½ cup veggie stock
- 1 tablespoon cilantro, chopped

Directions:

1. Heat up a pan with the oil over medium heat, add the shallots and the garlic and cook for 5 minutes.
2. Add the kale and the other ingredients, toss, cook for 15 minutes more, divide between plates and serve.

Nutrition:

calories 191, fat 7, fiber 3.5, carbs 28.1, protein 7.5

Radish and Cabbage

Prep time: 5 minutes | **Cooking time:** 20 minutes | **Servings:** 2

Ingredients:

- 1 green cabbage head, shredded
- 1 cup radishes, halved
- 2 scallions, chopped
- 2 tablespoons avocado oil
- ½ teaspoon garlic powder
- 1 teaspoon sweet paprika
- 1 tablespoon cilantro, chopped

Directions:

1. Heat up a pan with the oil over medium heat, add the scallions and garlic powder and cook for 5 minutes.
2. Add the cabbage and the other ingredients, toss, cook for 15 minutes more, divide between plates and serve.

Nutrition:

calories 127, fat 2.4, fiber 11.5, carbs 25.3, protein 5.7

Chives Cauliflower

Prep time: 5 minutes | **Cooking time:** 15 minutes | **Servings:** 2

Ingredients:

- ¼ cup veggie stock
- 1 pound cauliflower florets
- 1 tablespoon avocado oil
- 2 garlic cloves, minced
- 1 teaspoon hot paprika
- A pinch of salt and black pepper
- 1 tablespoon chives, chopped

Directions:

1. Heat up a pan with the oil over medium heat, add the garlic and the paprika and cook for 2 minutes.
2. Add the cauliflower and the other ingredients, toss, cook for 13 minutes, divide between plates and serve as a side dish.

Nutrition:

calories 71, fat 1.2, fiber 6.1, carbs 13.4, protein 4.8

Scallions Zucchini

Prep time: 5 minutes | **Cooking time:** 10 minutes | **Servings:** 2

Ingredients:

- 2 zucchinis, sliced
- 3 scallions, chopped
- 2 garlic cloves, minced
- 1 tablespoon rosemary, chopped
- 1 tablespoon olive oil
- 1 tablespoon balsamic vinegar
- A pinch of salt and black pepper
- ½ teaspoon sweet paprika

Directions:

1. Heat up a pan with the oil over medium heat, add the scallions and garlic and cook for 2 minutes.
2. Add the zucchinis and the other ingredients, toss, cook for 8 minutes more, divide between plates and serve.

Nutrition:

calories 112, fat 7.7, fiber 3.7, carbs 10.7, protein 3.1

Baby Spinach Saute

Prep time: 5 minutes | **Cooking time:** 15 minutes | **Servings:** 2

Ingredients:

- 1 pound baby spinach
- 1 tablespoon avocado oil
- 2 scallions, chopped
- 2 garlic cloves, minced
- 1 tablespoon lime juice
- A pinch of salt and black pepper

Direction:

1. Heat up a pan with the oil over medium heat, add the scallions and the garlic and cook for 5 minutes.
2. Add the spinach and the other ingredients, toss, cook for 10 minutes, divide between plates and serve.

Nutrition:

calories 135, fat 11, fiber 4, carbs 6, protein 3

Marinated Cucumbers

Prep time: 5 minutes | **Servings:** 2

Ingredients:

- ½ pound cucumbers, sliced
- 4 scallions, chopped
- 1 tablespoon olive oil
- 1 tablespoon balsamic vinegar
- A pinch of salt and black pepper
- 1 tablespoon dill, chopped

Directions:

1. 1. In a bowl, combine the cucumbers with the scallions and the other ingredients, toss, divide everything between plates and serve.

Nutrition:

calories 70, fat 3, fiber 2, carbs 6, protein 4

Cumin Stew

Prep time: 5 minutes | **Cooking time:** 20 minutes | **Servings:** 2

Ingredients:

- 2 shallots, chopped
- 1 teaspoon cumin, ground
- 1 red bell pepper, cut into strips
- 1 green bell pepper, cut into strips
- 1 orange bell pepper, cut into strips
- 1 tablespoon rosemary, chopped
- 2 tablespoons lime juice
- 1 tablespoon olive oil
- A pinch of salt and black pepper

Directions:

1. Heat up a pan with the oil over medium heat, add the shallots and sauté for 5 minutes.
2. Add the peppers and the other ingredients, stir, cook for 15 minutes, divide everything between plates and serve.

Nutrition:

calories 300, fat 32, fiber 7, carbs 6, protein 8

Lime Taste Salad

Prep time: 5 minutes | **Servings:** 2

Ingredients:

- 2 cups baby arugula
- 1 cup black olives, pitted and halved
- ½ cup cucumbers, sliced
- 1 tablespoon olive oil
- 2 tablespoons lime juice
- A pinch of salt and black pepper

Directions:

1. 1. In a bowl, combine the olives with the arugula and the other ingredients, toss and serve as a side dish.

Nutrition:

calories 160, fat 4, fiber 2, carbs 2, protein 6

Sliced Cucumbers and Cabbage Salad

Prep time: 10 minutes | **Servings:** 2

Ingredients:

- 2 cucumbers, sliced
- 1 tablespoon olive oil
- Juice of 1 lime
- 1 tablespoon dill, chopped
- 1 green cabbage head, shredded
- A pinch of salt and black pepper
- 1 garlic clove, minced
- 1 tablespoon cilantro, chopped

Directions:

1. 1. In a bowl, combine the cucumbers with the cabbage and the other ingredients, toss and serve as a side salad.

Nutrition:

calories 90, fat 0, fiber 2, carbs 2, protein 4

Dill Zoodles

Prep time: 5 minutes | **Cooking time:** 10 minutes | **Servings:** 2

Ingredients:

- 3 zucchinis, cut with a spiralizer
- 1 tablespoon capers, drained
- 1 tablespoon olive oil
- 1 tablespoon balsamic vinegar
- 2 garlic cloves, minced
- 1 tablespoon dill, chopped
- A pinch of salt and black pepper

Directions:

1. 1. Heat up a pan with the oil over medium heat, add the zucchinis and the other ingredients, toss, cook for 10 minutes, divide between plates and serve as a side dish.

Nutrition:

calories 100, fat 2, fiber 2, carbs 1, protein 9

Fennel Bulb Salad

Prep time: 10 minutes | **Servings:** 2

Ingredients:

- ½ pound cherry tomatoes, halved
- 1 fennel bulb, shredded
- 1 tablespoon lime juice
- 1 tablespoon olive oil
- 1 tablespoon pine nuts, toasted
- 1 tablespoon dill, chopped
- A pinch of salt and black pepper

Directions:

1. 1. In a bowl, mix the tomatoes with the fennel and the other ingredients, toss and serve as a side salad.

Nutrition:

calories 80, fat 0.2, fiber 1, carbs 0.4, protein 5

Keto Avocado Bowl

Prep time: 5 minutes | **Servings:** 4

Ingredients:

- 1 cup baby arugula
- 1 avocado, peeled, pitted and cubed
- 1 cup kalamata olives, pitted and halved
- 1 tablespoon olive oil
- 2 shallots, chopped
- 1 tablespoon chives, chopped
- A pinch of salt and black pepper

Directions:

1. 1. In a bowl, combine the arugula with the avocado and the other ingredients, toss and serve.

Nutrition:

calories 120, fat 3, fiber 2, carbs 1, protein 8

Flaked Red Pepper Mushrooms

Prep time: 5 minutes | **Cooking time:** 20 minutes | **Servings:** 2

Ingredients:

- 1 pound mushrooms, halved
- 1 tablespoon olive oil
- 3 scallions, chopped
- 1 teaspoon chili powder
- 3 garlic cloves, minced
- A pinch of salt and black pepper
- 1 tablespoon red pepper flakes, crushed
- 1 tablespoon chives, chopped

Directions:

1. Heat up a pan with the oil over medium heat, add the scallions, garlic and the chili powder and cook for 5 minutes.
2. Add the mushrooms and the other ingredients, toss, cook for 15 minutes more, divide the mix between plates and serve as a side dish.

Nutrition:

calories 143, fat 3, fiber 4, carbs 3, protein 4.6

Zucchini Medley

Prep time: 5 minutes | **Cooking time:** 20 minutes | **Servings:** 2

Ingredients:

- 1 cup cherry tomatoes, halved
- 1 cup zucchini, cubed
- 1 cup black olives, pitted and halved
- 1 avocado, peeled, pitted and cubed
- 2 garlic cloves, minced
- 1 cup baby spinach
- 2 tablespoons olive oil
- 1 tablespoon lime juice
- 1 tablespoon rosemary, chopped
- 1 tablespoon balsamic vinegar
- A pinch of salt and black pepper

Directions:

1. Heat up a pan with the oil over medium heat, add the garlic and garam masala, stir and cook for 2 minutes.
2. Add the cherry tomatoes and the other ingredients, toss, cook everything for 18 minutes more, divide between plates and serve as a side dish.

Nutrition:

calories 150, fat 1, fiber 2, carbs 1, protein 8

Hemp Seeds Mushrooms

Prep time: 10 minutes | **Cooking time:** 20 minutes | **Servings:** 2

Ingredients:

- 2 tablespoons ghee, melted
- 1 pound mushrooms, halved
- 2 garlic cloves, minced
- 1 cup cherry tomatoes, halved
- 1 cup kalamata olives, pitted and halved
- 1 cup hemp seeds
- A pinch of salt and black pepper
- ½ teaspoon garlic powder
- Juice of ½ lime
- ¼ tablespoon parsley, chopped

Directions:

1. Heat up a pan with the ghee over medium heat, add the garlic and the mushrooms and cook for 5 minutes.
2. Add the tomatoes and the other ingredients, toss, cook for 15 minutes more, divide between plates and serve.

Nutrition:

calories 324, fat 24, fiber 15, carbs 2, protein 15

Spiced Vegetables

Prep time: 5 minutes | **Cooking time:** 14 minutes | **Servings:** 2

Ingredients:

- 1 pound radishes, halved
- ½ red onion, chopped
- 3 scallions, chopped
- 1 tablespoon olive oil
- 1 teaspoon mustard
- 1 tablespoon balsamic vinegar
- 2 tablespoons olive oil
- Salt and black pepper to the taste

Directions:

1. Heat up a pan with the oil over medium heat, add the onion and the scallions and cook for 4 minutes.
2. Add the radishes and the other ingredients, toss, cook the mix for 10 minutes more, divide the mix between plates and serve.

Nutrition:

calories 140, fat 1, fiber 2, carbs 1, protein 7

Green Chili Pepper Tomatoes

Prep time: 10 minutes | **Servings:** 2

Ingredients:

- 1 pound cherry tomatoes, halved
- 2 tablespoons mint, chopped
- Juice of 1 lime
- 1 tablespoon olive oil
- 2 garlic cloves, minced
- Salt and black pepper to the taste
- 1 green chili pepper, seedless

Directions:

1. 1. In a bowl, combine the tomatoes with the mint, the oil and the other ingredients, toss and serve.

Nutrition:

calories 100, fat 1, fiber 1, carbs 0.4, protein 6

Sage Zucchini

Prep time: 5 minutes | **Cooking time:** 15 minutes | **Servings:** 2

Ingredients:

- 1 pound zucchinis, roughly cubed
- ½ teaspoon garam masala
- 1 tablespoon olive oil
- 1 tablespoon sage, chopped
- ½ teaspoon fennel seeds
- ½ teaspoon cayenne pepper
- ½ teaspoon sweet paprika

Directions:

1. 1. Heat up a pan with the oil over medium heat, add the zucchinis, garam masala and the other ingredients, toss, cook for 15 minutes, divide between plates and serve.

Nutrition:

calories 120, fat 1, fiber 3, carbs 5, protein 9

Lime and Vinegar Cauliflower

Prep time: 5 minutes | **Cooking time:** 20 minutes | **Servings:** 2

Ingredients:

- 1 pound cauliflower florets
- 3 garlic cloves, minced
- Zest of 1 lime, grated
- 1 tablespoon balsamic vinegar
- 1 tablespoon olive oil
- A pinch of salt and black pepper
- 1 tablespoon chives, chopped

Directions:

1. In a roasting pan, combine the cauliflower with the garlic and the other ingredients, toss, and cook at 400 degrees F for 20 minutes.
2. Divide between plates and serve hot as a side dish.

Nutrition:

calories 55, fat 1, fiber 1, carbs 0.5, protein 7

Tender Zucchini Rice

Prep time: 10 minutes | **Cooking time:** 20 minutes | **Servings:** 2

Ingredients:

- 1 zucchini, cubed
- 1 cup cauliflower rice
- 2 cups chicken broth
- 1 tablespoon olive oil
- 2 scallions, chopped
- 1 teaspoon chili powder
- ½ teaspoon red pepper flakes, crushed
- 1 red chili pepper, minced
- 4 green onions, chopped

Directions:

1. Heat up a pan with the oil over medium heat, add the scallions, chili powder, pepper flakes and chili pepper, stir and cook for 5 minutes.
2. Add the zucchini, rice and the other ingredients, toss, cook for 15 minutes more, divide between plates and serve.

Nutrition:

calories 142, fat 7, fiber 4, carbs 5, protein 3

Mustard Seeds Kale

Prep time: 5 minutes | **Cooking time:** 15 minutes | **Servings:** 2

Ingredients:

- 1-pound kale, torn
- 2 green chilies, minced
- 2 curry leaves, minced
- 1 tablespoon olive oil
- 3 scallions, chopped
- A pinch of salt and black pepper
- 2 garlic cloves, minced
- ¼ teaspoon mustard seeds, crushed
- 1 tablespoon chives, chopped

Directions:

1. Heat up a pan with the oil over medium heat, add the scallions and the garlic and cook for 2 minutes.
2. Add the kale and the other ingredients, toss, cook for 13 minutes more, divide between plates and serve.

Nutrition:

calories 90, fat 1, fiber 1, carbs 1, protein 6

Tarragon Fennel

Prep time: 5 minutes | **Cooking time:** 20 minutes | **Servings:** 2

Ingredients:

- 2 fennel bulbs, sliced
- 1 tablespoon shallots, chopped
- 1 tablespoon balsamic vinegar
- 2 tablespoons olive oil
- ½ cup coconut cream
- 1 tablespoon chives, chopped
- A pinch of salt and black pepper
- 1 tablespoon tarragon, chopped
- 1 tablespoon chives, chopped

Directions:

1. Heat up a pan with the oil over medium heat, add the shallots and cook for 2 minutes.
2. Add the fennel and the other ingredients, toss, cook for 18 minutes more, divide between plates and serve as a side dish.

Nutrition:

calories 200, fat 3, fiber 5, carbs 2, protein 10

Tender Radish Stew

Prep time: 5 minutes | **Cooking time:** 15 minutes | **Servings:** 2

Ingredients:

- ½ pound radishes, halved
- 2 green onions, chopped
- 1 tablespoon avocado oil
- 2 garlic cloves, minced
- ½ teaspoon sweet paprika
- ½ teaspoon chili powder
- ½ cup chicken broth
- A pinch of salt and black pepper
- 1 tablespoon chives, minced

Directions:

1. Heat up a pan with the oil over medium high heat, add the green onions, garlic, paprika and chili powder and sauté for 2 minutes.
2. Add the radishes and the other ingredients, toss, cook the mix for 13 minutes more, divide between plates and serve.

Nutrition:

calories 43, fat 1.4, fiber 3, carbs 7.3, protein 1.7

Classic Keto Bowl

Prep time: 10 minutes | **Cooking time:** 15 minutes | **Serving:** 2

Ingredients:

- ½ pound green beans, trimmed and halved
- 1 garlic clove, minced
- 1 tablespoon lemon juice
- 2 teaspoons smoked paprika
- 1 tablespoon olive oil
- 1 tablespoon walnuts, chopped
- 1 tablespoon pine nuts, toasted
- ½ teaspoon sesame seeds
- ¼ teaspoon coriander, ground
- A pinch of salt and black pepper

Directions:

1. Heat up a pan with the oil over medium heat, add the garlic and the paprika and cook for 2 minutes.
2. Add the green beans and the other ingredients, toss, and cook for 13 minutes more.
3. Divide between plates and serve.

Nutrition:

calories 160, fat 12, fiber 4, carbs 6, protein 4

Cayenne Pepper Cauli

Prep time: 5 minutes | **Cooking time:** 20 minutes | **Servings:** 2

Ingredients:

- 1 cup cauliflower rice
- 2 cups chicken broth
- 2 scallions, chopped
- 2 tablespoons ghee, melted
- 1 tablespoon thyme, chopped
- 1 teaspoon sweet paprika
- A pinch of salt and black pepper
- A pinch of cayenne pepper
- ¼ cup chives, chopped

Directions:

1. Heat up a pan with the ghee over medium heat, add the scallions and cook for 2 minutes.
2. Add the rice, stock and the other ingredients, toss, cook for 18 minutes more, divide between plates and serve as a side dish.

Nutrition:

calories 208, fat 23, fiber 1, carbs 3.3, protein 14

Rosemary Peppers

Prep time: 5 minutes | **Cooking time:** 20 minutes | **Servings:** 2

Ingredients:
- 1 tablespoon olive oil
- 1 pound red bell peppers, cut into strips
- ½ teaspoon chili powder
- ½ teaspoon rosemary, dried
- 2 scallions, chopped
- 1 tablespoon balsamic vinegar
- Salt and black pepper to the taste

Directions:
1. Heat up a pan with the oil over medium heat, add the scallions and cook for 5 minutes.
2. Add the peppers and the other ingredients, toss, cook for 15 minutes more, divide between plates and serve as a keto side dish.

Nutrition:
calories 97, fat 4, fiber 2, carbs 6, protein 2

Mustard Greens and Olives

Prep time: 5 minutes | **Cooking time:** 20 minutes | **Servings:** 2

Ingredients:
- ½ pound mustard greens
- 1 tablespoon olive oil
- 1 cup black olives, pitted and halved
- 1 cup kalamata olives, pitted and halved
- 1 tablespoon capers, drained
- 1 tablespoon balsamic vinegar
- A pinch of salt and black pepper
- 1 tablespoon chives, chopped

Directions:
1. 1. Heat up a pan with the oil over medium heat, add the mustard greens, olives and the other ingredients, toss, cook for 20 minutes, divide between plates and serve as a side dish.

Nutrition:
calories 119, fat 7, fiber 3, carbs 7, protein 2

Baby Arugula Salad

Prep time: 10 minutes | **Servings:** 2

Ingredients:
- 2 cups baby spinach
- 1 cup baby arugula
- 1 cup cherry tomatoes, halved
- 2 scallions, chopped
- ½ cup kalamata olives, pitted and halved
- 1 tablespoon balsamic vinegar
- 2 tablespoons olive oil
- A pinch of salt and black pepper

Directions:
1. 1. In a bowl, combine the spinach with the arugula and the other ingredients, toss and serve as a side salad.

Nutrition:
calories 170, fat 11, fiber 3, carbs 7, protein 7

Fragrant Scallions

Prep time: 10 minutes | **Cooking time:** 10 minutes | **Servings:** 2

Ingredients:
- 2 endives, trimmed and shredded
- 1 tablespoon olive oil
- 1 tablespoon lime juice
- 4 scallions, chopped
- A pinch of salt and black pepper
- 1 tablespoon rosemary, chopped

Directions:
1. Heat up a pan with the oil over medium heat, add the scallions and cook for 2 minutes.
2. Add the endives and the other ingredients, toss, cook for 8 minutes more, divide between plates and serve.

Nutrition:
calories 150, fat 3, fiber 2, carbs 2, protein 7

Dill and Cucumber Bowl

Prep time: 5 minutes | **Servings:** 2

Ingredients:
- 2 cucumbers, sliced
- 1 cup radishes, halved
- 2 tablespoons avocado oil
- 1 tablespoon balsamic vinegar
- ¼ teaspoon red pepper flakes
- Salt and black pepper to the taste
- 1 tablespoon chives, chopped
- 1 tablespoon dill, chopped

Directions:
1. 1. In a bowl, combine the cucumbers with the radishes and the other ingredients, toss and serve.

Nutrition:
calories 400, fat 34, fiber 2, carbs 4, protein 2

Green Mushrooms

Prep time: 5 minutes | **Cooking time:** 12 minutes | **Servings:** 2

Ingredients:
- ½ pound mushrooms, sliced
- 1 cup broccoli florets
- 2 tablespoons olive oil
- A pinch of salt and black pepper
- 2 garlic cloves, minced
- 2 spring onions, chopped
- 3 ounces spinach, torn
- 2 tablespoons garlic, minced
- 1 tablespoon almonds, chopped

Directions:
1. Heat up a pan with the oil over medium high heat, add the onions and garlic and cook for 2 minutes.
2. Add the mushrooms and the other ingredients, toss, cook for 10 minutes, divide between plates and serve as a side dish.

Nutrition:
calories 247, fat 23, fiber 4, carbs 3, protein 7

Hot Cauli Rice

Prep time: 10 minutes | **Cooking time:** 20 minutes | **Servings:** 2

Ingredients:
- 1 cup cauliflower rice
- 2 cups chicken broth
- 2 scallions, chopped
- 2 tablespoons ghee, melted
- 2 garlic cloves, minced
- 1 teaspoon chili powder
- ½ teaspoon hot paprika
- 1 tablespoon cilantro, chopped

Directions:
1. Heat up a pan with the ghee over medium heat, add the scallions and the garlic and cook for 2 minutes.
2. Add the cauliflower rice and the other ingredients, toss, cook for 18 minutes more divide between plates and serve.

Nutrition:
calories 142, fat 21, fiber 12, carbs 3, protein 14

Tender Red Cabbage

Prep time: 5 minutes | **Cooking time:** 15 minutes | **Servings:** 2

Ingredients:
- 1 red cabbage head, shredded
- 3 scallions, minced
- Salt and black pepper to the taste
- 2 tablespoons ghee, melted
- 1 cup cherry tomatoes, halved
- 2 red chili peppers, minced
- ½ teaspoon sweet paprika
- 1 tablespoon chives, chopped

Directions:
1. Heat up a pan with the ghee over medium heat, add the scallions, chili peppers and the paprika and cook for 2 minutes.
2. Add the cabbage and the other ingredients, toss, cook for 13 minutes more, divide the mix between plates and serve.

Nutrition:
calories 200, fat 4, fiber 2, carbs 3, protein 7

Aromatic Keto Mix

Prep time: 5 minutes | **Cooking time:** 15 minutes | **Servings:** 2

Ingredients:

- 1 tablespoon olive oil
- ½ pound cherry tomatoes, halved
- ¼ cup shallots, minced
- 2 garlic cloves, minced
- 1 pound green beans, trimmed and halved
- 2 tablespoons pine nuts
- 1 tablespoon rosemary, chopped
- A pinch of salt and black pepper

Directions:

1. Heat up a pan with the oil over medium heat, add the shallots and the garlic and cook for 2 minutes.
2. Add the green beans and the other ingredients, toss, cook for 13 minutes more, divide between plates and serve as a side dish.

Nutrition:

calories 233, fat 13.7, fiber 10.2, carbs 27.1, protein 7.1

Herbs de Provence Olives

Prep time: 10 minutes | **Cooking time:** 10 minutes | **Servings:** 2

Ingredients:

- 1 cup black olives, pitted
- 1 cup kalamata olives, pitted
- 1 cup green olives, pitted
- 2 scallions, chopped
- 1 tablespoon olive oil
- 1 tablespoon chives, chopped
- 1 tablespoon oregano, chopped
- 1 tablespoon herbes de Provence
- A pinch of salt and black pepper

Directions:

1. Heat up a pan with the oil over medium heat, add the scallions and cook for 2 minutes.
2. Add the olives and the other ingredients, toss, cook for 8 minutes more, divide between plates and serve.

Nutrition:

calories 200, fat 20, fiber 4, carbs 3, protein 1

Jalapeno and Cheddar Cheese Mix

Prep time: 10 minutes | **Cooking time:** 20 minutes | **Servings:** 2

Ingredients:

- 1 pound cherry tomatoes, halved
- 1 tablespoon olive oil
- 3 scallions, chopped
- ½ cup cheddar cheese, shredded
- 1 tablespoon jalapeno pepper, chopped
- Salt and black pepper to the taste
- 2 tablespoons cilantro, chopped

Directions:

1. In a baking dish, combine the tomatoes with the oil, scallions and the other ingredients except the cheese and toss.
2. Sprinkle the cheese on top, introduce the pan in the oven and cook at 380 degrees F for 20 minutes.
3. Divide between plates and serve

Nutrition:

calories 260, fat 22, fiber 4, carbs 3, protein 10

Soft and Aromatic Radish Bowl

Prep time: 10 minutes | **Cooking time:** 10 minutes | **Servings:** 2

Ingredients:

- 1 pound radishes, halved
- 1 cup kalamata olives, pitted and halved
- 2 tablespoons ghee, melted
- 1 tablespoons parsley, chopped
- 1 tablespoon mustard
- A pinch of salt and black pepper
- ½ teaspoon turmeric powder
- 2 garlic cloves, minced

Directions:

1. 1. Heat up a pan with the ghee over medium heat, add the radishes, olives and the other ingredients, toss, cook for 10 minutes, divide between plates and serve as a side dish.

Nutrition:

calories 87, fat 2.4, fiber 3, carbs 5, protein 4

Cumin and Oregano Radish

Prep time: 5 minutes | **Cooking time:** 12 minutes | **Servings:** 2

Ingredients:

- 2 tablespoons ghee, melted
- 1 pound radishes, halved
- 1 teaspoon garlic powder
- 1 tablespoon oregano, chopped
- 1 teaspoon onion powder
- 1 teaspoon cumin, ground
- 1 tablespoon chives, chopped

Directions:

1. 1. Heat up a pan with the ghee over medium heat, add the radishes and the other ingredients, toss, cook for 12 minutes, divide between plates and serve.

Nutrition:

calories 140, fat 2, fiber 1, carbs 1, protein 6

Indian Style Cauliflower

Prep time: 10 minutes | **Cooking time:** 20 minutes | **Servings:** 2

Ingredients:

- 1 cup cauliflower florets
- 1 cup broccoli florets
- 1 tablespoon sweet paprika
- 1 teaspoon garam masala
- 2 tablespoons ghee, melted
- Salt and black pepper to the taste
- ½ tablespoon cilantro, chopped

Directions:

1. 1. Heat up a pan with the ghee over medium heat, add the cauliflower, broccoli and the other ingredients, toss, cook for 20 minutes, divide between plates and serve as a side dish.

Nutrition:

calories 190, fat 16, fiber 7, carbs 3, protein 5

Rosemary Mushroom Rice

Prep time: 10 minutes | **Cooking time:** 25 minutes | **Servings:** 2

Ingredients:

- 1 cup cauliflower rice
- ½ cup mushrooms, halved
- 1 tablespoon olive oil
- 2 cups chicken broth
- ½ teaspoon turmeric powder
- ½ teaspoon rosemary, dried
- 2 scallions, chopped
- A pinch of salt and black pepper

Directions:

1. Heat up a pan with the oil over medium heat, add the scallions and the mushrooms and cook for 5 minutes.
2. Add the cauliflower rice and the other ingredients, toss, cook for 20 minutes more, divide between plates and serve as a side dish.

Nutrition:

calories 345, fat 34, fiber 0, carbs 2, protein 4

Coconut Cream and Cumin Radish Mix

Prep time: 10 minutes | **Cooking time:** 12 minutes | **Servings:** 2

Ingredients:

- 1 pound radishes, halved
- 1 tablespoon olive oil
- 2 scallions, chopped
- ½ teaspoon cumin, ground
- ½ teaspoon coriander, ground
- 1 cup coconut cream
- 1 tablespoon parsley, chopped
- 1 jalapeno pepper, chopped
- A pinch of salt and black pepper

Directions:

1. Heat up a pan with the oil over medium heat, add the scallions and cook for 2 minutes.
2. Add the radishes and the other ingredients, toss, cook for 10 minutes more, divide between plates and serve as a side dish.

Nutrition:

calories 340, fat 4, fiber 6, carbs 3.4, protein 7

Cumin Kale

Prep time: 5 minutes | **Cooking time:** 20 minutes | **Servings:** 2

Ingredients:

- 1 pound kale, torn
- 1 cup radishes, halved
- 3 garlic cloves, minced
- Juice of 1 lime
- 2 tablespoons olive oil
- A pinch of salt and black pepper
- ¼ teaspoon cumin, ground
- ½ teaspoon basil, dried

Directions:

1. Heat up a pan with the oil over medium heat, add the garlic and cook for 2 minutes.
2. Add the kale, radish and the other ingredients, toss, cook for 18 minutes more, divide between plates and serve.

Nutrition:

calories 249, fat 14.1, fiber 4.5, carbs 27.5, protein 7.5

Aromatic Brussel Sprouts

Prep time: 5 minutes | **Cooking time:** 20 minutes | **Servings:** 2

Ingredients:

- 2 shallots, chopped
- 2 garlic cloves, minced
- ½ pound Brussels sprouts, trimmed and halved
- 1 tablespoon olive oil
- ½ cup veggie stock
- ½ teaspoon chili powder
- 1 tablespoon cilantro, chopped
- A pinch of salt and black pepper

Directions:

1. Heat up a pan with the oil over medium heat, add the garlic and the shallots and cook for 5 minutes.
2. Add the sprouts, stock and the other ingredients, toss, cook for 15 minutes more, divide between plates and serve as a side dish.

Nutrition:

calories 116, fat 7.5, fiber 4.6, carbs 11.7, protein 4.2

Fragrant Mushrooms

Prep time: 5 minutes | **Cooking time:** 20 minutes | **Servings:** 4

Ingredients:

- 1 pound mushrooms, halved
- 3 garlic cloves, minced
- 1 tablespoon rosemary, chopped
- 1 tablespoon olive oil
- ½ teaspoon sweet paprika
- A pinch of salt and black pepper
- ¼ cup veggie stock

Directions:

1. Heat up a pan with the oil over medium high heat, add the garlic and the paprika and cook for 2 minutes.
2. Add the mushrooms and the other ingredients, toss, cook everything for 18 minutes more, divide between plates and serve as a side dish.

Nutrition:

calories 70, fat 1, fiber 1, carbs 0.4, protein 6

Cumin Green Beans

Prep time: 5 minutes | **Cooking time:** 20 minutes | **Servings:** 4

Ingredients:

- 1 pound green beans, trimmed
- ½ cup cheddar cheese, shredded
- 2 tablespoons lime juice
- 1 tablespoon avocado oil
- A pinch of salt and black pepper
- 1 teaspoon sweet paprika
- ½ teaspoon cumin, ground
- 1 tablespoon chives, chopped

Directions:

1. In a roasting pan, combine the green beans with the lime juice and the other ingredients except the cheese and toss.
2. Sprinkle the cheese on top, bake at 400 degrees F for 20 minutes, divide everything between plates and serve as a side dish.

Nutrition:

calories 170, fat 15, fiber 4, carbs 4, protein 4

Parmesan Radishes

Prep time: 10 minutes | **Cooking time:** 20 minutes | **Servings:** 2

Ingredients:

- 1 pound radishes, halved
- 2 garlic cloves, minced
- 1 tablespoon olive oil
- Juice of ½ lime
- 2 shallots, chopped
- ¼ cup parmesan, grated
- 1 tablespoon chives, chopped
- A pinch of salt and black pepper

Directions:

1. In a roasting pan, combine the radishes with the garlic and the other ingredients, toss, introduce the oven and bake at 390 degrees F for 20 minutes.
2. Divide the mix between plates and serve.

Nutrition:

calories 193, fat 14, fiber 3, carbs 6, protein 5

Kalamata Olives and Fennel

Prep time: 10 minutes | **Cooking time:** 10 minutes | **Servings:** 2

Ingredients:

- 2 fennel bulbs, sliced
- ½ cup black olives, pitted and halved
- ½ cup kalamata olives, pitted and halved
- 1 tablespoon olive oil
- Salt and black pepper to the taste
- 5 scallions, chopped
- A handful cilantro, chopped

Directions:

1. Heat up a pan with the oil over medium heat, add the scallions and cook for 2 minutes.
2. Add the fennel and the other ingredients, toss, cook for 8 minutes more, divide between plates and serve.

Nutrition:

calories 123, fat 11.2, fiber 2.3, carbs 4.5, protein 4

Dill Mix

Prep time: 10 minutes | **Servings:** 2

Ingredients:

- 1 cup black olives, pitted and halved
- 1 cup green olives, pitted and halved
- 1 cup kalamata olives, pitted and halved
- ½ cup cherry tomatoes, cubed
- 1 tablespoon olive oil
- 1 tablespoon balsamic vinegar
- 1 tablespoon dill, chopped
- A pinch of salt and black pepper
- 1 tablespoons chives, chopped

Directions:

1. 1. In a bowl, combine the olives with the tomatoes, oil and the other ingredients, toss and serve as a side salad.

Nutrition:

calories 200, fat 2, fiber 2, carbs 1, protein 10

Dijon Mustard Mix

Prep time: 5 minutes | **Cooking time:** 10 minutes | **Servings:** 2

Ingredients:

- 2 avocados, peeled, pitted and roughly cubed
- 1 tablespoon garlic, minced
- 1 tablespoon olive oil
- 1 tablespoon Dijon mustard
- 1 tablespoon chives, chopped
- A pinch of salt and black pepper
- 1 tablespoon dill, chopped

Directions:

1. Heat up a pan with the oil over medium heat, add the garlic and cook for 2 minutes.
2. Add the avocados and the other ingredients, toss, cook for 8 minutes more, divide between plates and serve.

Nutrition:

calories 70, fat 4, fiber 2, carbs 4, protein 2.4

Keto Caps

Prep time: 10 minutes | **Cooking time:** 25 minutes | **Servings:** 2

Ingredients:

- 1-pound baby Bella mushroom caps
- A pinch of salt and black pepper
- 2 tablespoons shallots, chopped
- 2 garlic cloves, minced
- 3 tablespoons parsley flakes
- 1 teaspoon garlic powder

Directions:

1. In a roasting pan, combine the mushroom caps with the shallots and the other ingredients, toss and cook at 380 degrees F for 25 minutes.
2. Divide between plates and serve.

Nutrition:

calories 152, fat 12, fiber 5, carbs 6, protein 4

Chili Powder Salad

Prep time: 5 minutes | **Cooking time:** 15 minutes | **Servings:** 2

Ingredients:

- 1 cup cauliflower florets
- 1 cup cucumber, sliced
- 1 tablespoon olive oil
- Juice of 1 lime
- 1 teaspoon chili powder
- A pinch of salt and black pepper
- 1 teaspoon coriander, ground

Directions:

1. 1. Heat up a pan with the oil over medium heat, add the cauliflower, cucumber and the other ingredients, toss, cook for 15 minutes, divide between plates and serve.

Nutrition:

calories 211, fat 20, fiber 2, carbs 3, protein 4

Tender Ghee Rice

Prep time: 10 minutes | **Cooking time:** 20 minutes | **Servings:** 2

Ingredients:

- 1 cup cauliflower rice
- 1 cup chicken broth
- 1 cup coconut cream
- 2 scallions, chopped
- 2 tablespoons ghee, melted
- A pinch of salt and black pepper
- 1 tablespoon chives, chopped

Directions:

1. Heat up a pan with the ghee over medium heat, add the scallions and cook for 2 minutes.
2. Add the cauliflower rice and the other ingredients, toss, cook for 18 minutes more, divide between plates and serve as a side dish.

Nutrition:

calories 108, fat 3, fiber 6, carbs 5, protein 9

Cilantro and Vegetables Mix

Prep time: 10 minutes | **Cooking time:** 12 minutes | **Servings:** 2

Ingredients:

- 2 avocados, peeled, pitted and roughly cubed
- ½ pound Brussels sprouts, trimmed and halved
- 1 tablespoon lime juice
- 1 tablespoon olive oil
- ½ teaspoon chili powder
- A pinch of salt and black pepper
- ¼ cup cilantro, chopped
- 1 tablespoon chives, chopped

Directions:

1. 1. Heat up a pan with the oil over medium heat, add the sprouts, avocado and the other ingredients, toss, cook for 12 minutes, divide between plates and serve.

Nutrition:

calories 80, fat 1, fiber 2, carbs 1, protein 4

Cajun Seasonings and Keto Vegetables

Prep time: 10 minutes | **Cooking time:** 14 minutes | **Servings:** 2

Ingredients:

- 2 zucchinis, sliced
- 1 tablespoon olive oil
- Juice of 1 lime
- Zest of 1 lime, grated
- A pinch of salt and black pepper
- 1 teaspoon Cajun seasoning
- A pinch of cayenne pepper
- 1 tablespoon chives, chopped

Directions:

1. 1. Heat up a pan with the oil over medium heat, add the zucchinis, lime juice and the other ingredients, toss, cook for 14 minutes more, divide between plates and serve.

Nutrition:

calories 200, fat 2, fiber 1, carbs 5, protein 8

Herbs de Provence Olives

Prep time: 10 minutes | **Cooking time:** 10 minutes | **Servings:** 2

Ingredients:

- 1 cup black olives, pitted
- 1 cup kalamata olives, pitted
- 1 cup green olives, pitted
- 2 scallions, chopped
- 1 tablespoon olive oil
- 1 tablespoon chives, chopped
- 1 tablespoon oregano, chopped
- 1 tablespoon herbes de Provence
- A pinch of salt and black pepper

Directions:

1. Heat up a pan with the oil over medium heat, add the scallions and cook for 2 minutes.
2. Add the olives and the other ingredients, toss, cook for 8 minutes more, divide between plates and serve.

Nutrition:

calories 200, fat 20, fiber 4, carbs 3, protein 1

Caraway Seeds Mix of Vegetables

Prep time: 10 minutes | **Cooking time:** 14 minutes | **Servings:** 2

Ingredients:

- 2 tablespoons ghee, melted
- 2 zucchinis, sliced
- 1 red bell pepper, roughly cubed
- 1 green bell pepper, roughly cubed
- 1 teaspoon caraway seeds, crushed
- 1 teaspoon sweet paprika
- 1 cup coconut cream
- 1 tablespoon dill, chopped
- A pinch of salt and black pepper
- ¼ teaspoon cayenne pepper

Directions:

1. 1. Heat up a pan with the ghee over medium heat, add the zucchinis, bell peppers and the other ingredients, toss, cook for 14 minutes more, divide between plate and serve.

Nutrition:

calories 200, fat 13, fiber 0, carbs 1, protein 6

Chives Stew

Prep time: 10 minutes | **Cooking time:** 20 minutes | **Servings:** 2

Ingredients:

- 1 pound green beans, trimmed and halved
- 1 tablespoon olive oil
- ½ tablespoon lime zest, grated
- 1 red onion, chopped
- A pinch of salt and black pepper
- 1 tablespoon chives, chopped
- 3 garlic cloves, minced

Directions:

1. Heat up a pan with the oil over medium heat, add the onion and lime zest and cook for 5 minutes.
2. Add the green beans and the other ingredients, toss, cook for 15 minutes more, divide between plates and serve.

Nutrition:

calories 50, fat 1, fiber 1, carbs 6, protein 2

Ketogenic Snacks and Appetizers Recipes

Parsley Cheese Spread

Prep time: 10 minutes | **Servings:** 2

Ingredients:

- 3 ounces cream cheese
- ¼ teaspoon garlic powder
- 3 garlic cloves, minced
- 1 tablespoon chives, chopped
- ½ teaspoon turmeric powder
- Salt and black pepper to the taste
- 1 jalapeno pepper, chopped
- ½ teaspoon parsley, dried

Directions:

1. 1. In a blender, combine the cream cheese with the garlic and the other ingredients, pulse well, divide into bowls and serve cold as a party spread.

Nutrition:

calories 200, fat 18, fiber 1, carbs 2, protein 5

Mozzarella and Vegetables Dip

Prep time: 10 minutes | **Cooking time:** 20 minutes | **Servings:** 4

Ingredients:

- ½ cup mozzarella cheese
- 1 cup coconut cream
- 1 zucchini, cubed
- Salt and black pepper to the taste
- ½ teaspoon Italian seasoning
- 1 tablespoon cilantro, chopped

Directions:

1. In a ramekin, combine the cheese with the cream and the other ingredients, whisk well and cook at 390 degrees F for 20 minutes.
2. Serve the dip warm.

Nutrition:

calories 400, fat 34, fiber 4, carbs 4, protein 15

Kale and Scallions Salsa

Prep time: 10 minutes | **Cooking time:** 15 minutes | **Servings:** 2

Ingredients:

- 1 cup kale, torn
- 1 tablespoon olive oil
- 1 tablespoon lime juice
- 1 cup black olives, pitted and halved
- 1 avocado, peeled, pitted and cubed
- A pinch of salt and black pepper
- 2 scallions, chopped

Directions:

1. Heat up a pan with the oil over medium heat, add the scallions, kale and the other ingredients, toss and cook for 15 minutes.
2. Divide into bowls and serve as an appetizer.

Nutrition:

calories 80, fat 6, fiber 1, carbs 1, protein 3

Seeds and Nuts Snack

Prep time: 10 minutes | **Cooking time:** 10 minutes | **Servings:** 2

Ingredients:

- 1 cup black olives, pitted and halved
- 1 cup almonds, toasted
- 2 tablespoons sunflower seeds
- 1 tablespoon cilantro, chopped
- A pinch of red pepper flakes
- 1 and ½ tablespoons olive oil

Directions:

1. 1. Heat up a pan with the oil over medium heat, add the olives, almonds and the other ingredients, toss, cook for 10 minutes, divide into bowls and serve as a snack.

Nutrition:

calories 100, fat 43, fiber 4, carbs 2, protein 3

Ketogenic Seafood and Fish Recipes

Cumin Salmon

Prep time: 10 minutes | **Cooking time:** 20 minutes | **Servings:** 2

Ingredients:

- 2 shallots, minced
- 2 spring onions, chopped
- 2 tablespoons avocado oil
- 2 salmon fillets, boneless
- 1 tablespoon chives, chopped
- 1 teaspoon cumin, ground
- ½ teaspoon oregano, dried
- A pinch of salt and black pepper

Directions:

1. Heat up a pan with the oil over medium heat, add the shallots, spring onions and the cumin and cook for 5 minutes.
2. Add the fish and the other ingredients, cook the mix for 15 minutes, divide between plates and serve.

Nutrition:

calories 265, fat 13.1, fiber 1.4, carbs 2.7, protein 35.3

Meat Muffins

Prep time: 10 minutes | **Cooking time:** 30 minutes | **Servings:** 2

Ingredients:

- ½ cup almond flour
- A pinch of salt and black pepper
- 2 eggs
- 1 teaspoon baking powder
- ¼ cup coconut cream
- ½ teaspoon onion powder
- ½ pound beef, ground
- ½ teaspoon garlic powder
- ½ cup cheddar cheese, grated

Directions:

1. In a bowl, combine the beef with the flour, eggs and the other ingredients, stir well, divide into a muffin tray and cook at 390 degrees F fro 30 minutes.
2. Arrange the muffins on a platter and serve.

Nutrition:

calories 245, fat 16, fiber 6, carbs 2, protein 14

Turmeric Trout

Prep time: 10 minutes | **Cooking time:** 20 minutes | **Servings:** 2

Ingredients:

- 2 trout fillets, boneless
- 2 tablespoons lime zest
- 1 teaspoon turmeric powder
- 2 tablespoons olive oil
- A pinch of salt and black pepper
- ½ teaspoon lime juice

Directions:

1. 1. In a roasting pan, combine the trout with the turmeric, lime zest and the other ingredients, cook for 20 minutes at 390 degrees F, divide between plates and serve.

Nutrition:

calories 245, fat 19.7, fiber 0.9, carbs 1.7, protein 16.7

Oregano Dip

Prep time: 10 minutes | **Servings:** 2

Ingredients:

- 4 spring onions, chopped
- 1 tablespoon chives, chopped
- 1 tablespoon oregano, chopped
- 1 tablespoon basil, chopped
- 2 cups coconut cream
- A pinch of salt and black pepper

Directions:

1. 1. In a blender, combine the cream with the chives and the other ingredients, pulse well, divide into bowls and serve as a party dip.

Nutrition:

calories 569, fat 57.5, fiber 7.1, carbs 17.1, protein 6.4

Garlic Sea Bass

Prep time: 10 minutes | **Cooking time:** 20 minutes | **Servings:** 2

Ingredients:

- 2 sea fillets, boneless
- 2 tablespoons avocado oil
- 1 teaspoon chili powder
- 1 red chili, minced
- 1 teaspoon turmeric powder
- A pinch of salt and black pepper
- ¼ teaspoon garlic powder

Directions:

1. Heat up a pan with the oil over medium heat, add the chili, chili powder and turmeric and cook for 2 minutes.
2. Add the fish, and the other ingredients, cook for 18 minutes more, divide between plates and serve.

Nutrition:

calories 28, fat 2.1, fiber 1.4, carbs 2.5, protein 0.5

Lime Salmon

Prep time: 10 minutes | **Cooking time:** 15 minutes | **Servings:** 2

Ingredients:

- 2 salmon fillets, boneless
- Juice of 1 lime
- ½ cup shallots, chopped
- 2 tablespoons avocado oil
- A pinch of salt and black pepper
- 2 tablespoons walnuts, chopped

Directions:

1. Heat up a pan with the oil over medium high heat, add the shallots, stir and sauté for 5 minutes.
2. Add the fish and the other ingredients, cook for 10 minutes more, divide between plates and serve.

Nutrition:

calories 331, fat 17.4, fiber 1.2, carbs 8.7, protein 37.6

Tender Lemon Shrimp

Prep time: 5 minutes | **Cooking time:** 8 minutes | **Servings:** 2

Ingredients:

- ½ pound shrimp, peeled and deveined
- 1 tablespoon olive oil
- 2 shallots, chopped
- A pinch of salt and black pepper
- 3 tablespoons chives, chopped
- 1 tablespoon lemon juice

Directions:

1. Heat up a pan with the oil over medium heat, add the shallots and sauté for 2 minutes.
2. Add the shrimp and the other ingredients, toss, cook for 6 minutes more, divide between plates and serve.

Nutrition:

calories 198, fat 9, fiber 0.2, carbs 2.1, protein 26.1

Shrimps with Chicken broth

Prep time: 10 minutes | **Cooking time:** 10 minutes | **Servings:** 2

Ingredients:

- ½ pound shrimp, peeled and deveined
- 1 cup sun-dried tomatoes, chopped
- 1 tablespoon olive oil
- 2 spring onions, chopped
- ½ cup chicken broth
- A pinch of salt and black pepper
- ½ teaspoon basil, dried

Directions:

1. 1. Heat up a pan with the oil over medium heat, add the shrimp, tomatoes and the other ingredients, toss, cook for 10 minutes, divide into bowls and serve.

Nutrition:

calories 218, fat 9.3, fiber 1.5, carbs 6.5, protein 27.1

Radish Dip

Prep time: 10 minutes | **Servings:** 2

Ingredients:

- 1 cup radishes, chopped
- 6 ounces cream cheese, soft
- 1 tablespoon ghee, melted
- 1 tablespoon cilantro, chopped
- A pinch of cayenne pepper
- 1 teaspoon sweet paprika

Directions:

1. 1. In a blender, combine the radishes with the cream cheese and the other ingredients, pulse well, divide into small bowls and serve.

Nutrition:

calories 247, fat 25.4, fiber 1.1, carbs 3.3, protein 3.5

Walnuts Dip

Prep time: 10 minutes | **Servings:** 2

Ingredients:

- 1 cup walnuts, chopped
- 1 cup cream cheese, soft
- 1 tablespoon lime juice
- 1 tablespoon lime zest, grated
- A pinch of black pepper

Directions:

1. 1. In a blender, combine the cream cheese with the walnuts and the other ingredients, pulse well, divide into bowls and serve.

Nutrition:

calories 300, fat 13.4, fiber 1.2, carbs 6.2, protein 5

Pesto and Zucchini Dip

Prep time: 10 minutes | **Servings:** 2

Ingredients:

- 1 cup cream cheese, soft
- ½ cup zucchinis, grated
- 2 tablespoons basil pesto
- 2 tablespoons olive oil
- 2 tablespoons oregano, chopped
- 1 tablespoon chives, chopped
- A pinch of salt and black pepper

Directions:

1. 1. In a blender, combine the zucchinis with the cream cheese and the other ingredients, pulse well, divide into small bowls and serve.

Nutrition:

calories 150, fat 6.3, fiber 1, carbs 5.1, protein 2

Walnuts Snack Bowls

Prep time: 10 minutes | **Cooking time:** 20 minutes

Servings: 2

Ingredients:

- 1 teaspoon olive oil
- 1 cup walnuts
- ½ teaspoon cayenne pepper
- ½ teaspoon sweet paprika
- A pinch of salt and black pepper
- 1 tablespoon thyme, chopped

Directions:

1. Spread the walnuts on a baking sheet lined with parchment paper, add the oil and the other ingredients, toss and cook at 420 degrees F for 20 minutes.
- Divide into bowls and serve as a snack.

Nutrition:

calories 163, fat 13, fiber 1, carbs 5.3, protein 3

Lime Cream Dip

Prep time: 10 minutes | **Servings:** 2

Ingredients:

- Zest of 1 lime, grated
- 1 cup cream cheese, soft
- 1 cup coconut cream
- Juice of 1 lime
- A pinch of salt and black pepper
- ½ cup coconut oil, melted
- 1 tablespoon chives, chopped

Directions:

1. 1. In a blender, mix the cream cheese with the lime zest and the other ingredients, pulse well, divide into small cups and serve as a party dip.

Nutrition:

calories 150, fat 14, fiber 2, carbs 4, protein 2

Smoked Shrimp Platter

Prep time: 5 minutes | **Cooking time:** 12 minutes | **Servings:** 2

Ingredients:

- ½ pound shrimp, peeled and deveined
- 1 tablespoon olive oil
- 2 teaspoons smoked paprika
- A pinch of salt and black pepper
- 1 tablespoon lime juice

Directions:

1. Spread the shrimp on a baking sheet lined with parchment paper, add the oil and the other ingredients, toss and cook at 390 degrees F for 12 minutes.
2. Arrange the shrimp on a platter and serve.

Nutrition:

calories 245, fat 12, fiber 2, carbs 1, protein 14

Broccoli Bites

Prep time: 10 minutes | **Cooking time:** 20 minutes | **Servings:** 2

Ingredients:

- 1 cup broccoli florets
- 1 teaspoon sweet paprika
- A pinch of salt and black pepper
- Cooking spray
- 1 cup cheddar cheese, grated

Directions:

1. Arrange the broccoli on a baking sheet lined with parchment paper, add the paprika and the other ingredients, toss and bake at 380 degrees F for 20 minutes.
2. Serve as a snack.

Nutrition:

calories 163, fat 12, fiber 2, carbs 2, protein 7

Masala Dip

Prep time: 10 minutes | **Servings:** 4

Ingredients:

- 1 tablespoon olive oil
- 1 cup cream cheese, soft
- 1 cup coconut cream
- 1 teaspoon garam masala
- 1 tablespoon chives, chopped
- Salt and black pepper to the taste

Directions:

1. 1. In a blender, combine the cream cheese with the cream and the other ingredients, pulse well, divide into small cups and serve.

Nutrition:

calories 345, fat 33, fiber 4, carbs 5, protein 5

Peppers Salsa

Prep time: 10 minutes | **Servings:** 2

Ingredients:

- 1 pound red bell peppers, cubed
- 1 cup cherry tomatoes, halved
- 1 cup kalamata olives, pitted and halved
- A pinch of salt and black pepper
- 1 tablespoon olive oil
- Juice of 1 lime
- ½ teaspoon rosemary, dried
- 1 tablespoon chives, chopped

Directions:

1. 1. In a bowl, combine the peppers with the tomatoes and the other ingredients, toss, divide into small bowls and serve.

Nutrition:

calories 350, fat 22, fiber 3, carbs 6, protein 2

Seeds Snack

Prep time: 5 minutes | **Cooking time:** 20 minutes | **Servings:** 2

Ingredients:

- 1 cup sunflower seeds
- ½ cup walnuts, chopped
- 2 tablespoons olive oil
- A pinch of salt and black pepper
- ½ teaspoon coriander, ground

Directions:

1. Spread the sunflower seeds on a baking sheet lined with parchment paper, add the walnuts and the other ingredients, and toss.
2. Bake at 400 degrees F for 20 minutes, divide into bowls and serve as a snack.

Nutrition:

calories 140, fat 2, fiber 1, carbs 5, protein 1

Olives and Cream Cheese Spread

Prep time: 10 minutes | **Servings:** 4

Ingredients:

- 1 cup cream cheese, soft
- ½ cup black olives, pitted and chopped
- 1 tablespoon avocado oil
- 1 tablespoon basil, chopped
- ½ teaspoon rosemary, dried
- Salt and black pepper to the taste

Directions:

1. 1. In a blender, combine the cream cheese with the olive and the other ingredients, pulse well, divide into small bowls and serve.

Nutrition:

calories 140, fat 4, fiber 2, carbs 6, protein 4

Cucumbers Salsa

Prep time: 10 minutes | **Servings:** 2

Ingredients:

- 2 cups cherry tomatoes, halved
- 1 tablespoon olive oil
- Juice of 1 lime
- 3 spring onions, chopped
- 1 cup black olives, pitted and halved
- 1 cup cucumbers, cubed
- A pinch of salt and black pepper

Directions:

1. 1. In a bowl, combine the cherry tomatoes with the oil and the other ingredients, toss and serve as an appetizer.

Nutrition:

calories 40, fat 3, fiber 7, carbs 3, protein 7

Ghee and Garlic Spread

Prep time: 5 minutes | **Servings:** 2

Ingredients:

- 4 leeks, chopped
- 2 tablespoons ghee, melted
- 1 cup cream cheese, soft
- A pinch of salt and black pepper
- 4 garlic cloves, minced
- 1 tablespoon chives, chopped

Directions:

2. 1. In your blender, combine the leeks with the ghee and the other ingredients, pulse well, divide into bowls and serve cold.

Nutrition:

calories 80, fat 5, fiber 3, carbs 6, protein 7

Spring Onions Chicken Bites

Prep time: 6 minutes | **Cooking time:** 25 minutes | **Servings:** 2

Ingredients:

- ½ pound chicken breast, skinless, boneless and cubed
- 1 tablespoon olive oil
- 2 teaspoons sweet paprika
- 2 spring onions, chopped
- A pinch of salt and black pepper
- ½ teaspoon rosemary, dried

Directions:

1. In a bowl, mix the chicken with the oil and the other ingredients, toss, arrange the bites on a baking sheet lined with parchment paper and cook at 390 degrees F for 25 minutes.
2. Serve the bites as an appetizer.

Nutrition:

calories 100, fat 2, fiber 3, carbs 1, protein 6

Nutmeg Platter

Prep time: 10 minutes | **Cooking time:** 25 minutes | **Servings:** 2

Ingredients:

- 2 zucchinis, sliced
- ½ teaspoon nutmeg, ground
- ½ teaspoon cumin, ground
- ½ teaspoon coriander, ground
- ½ teaspoon turmeric powder
- 1 tablespoon olive oil
- Juice of 1 lime

Directions:

1. In a roasting pan, combine the zucchinis with the nutmeg, cumin and the other ingredients, toss and bake at 390 degrees F for 25 minutes.
2. Arrange the zucchinis on a platter and serve as an appetizer.

Nutrition:

calories 300, fat 12, fiber 4, carbs 3, protein 8

Poblano Peppers Dip

Prep time: 10 minutes | **Cooking time:** 20 minutes | **Servings:** 2

Ingredients:

- 1 cup shrimp, peeled, deveined, cooked and chopped
- 1 cup cream cheese, soft
- 1 tablespoon olive oil
- 1 tablespoon chives, chopped
- 2 poblano peppers, chopped
- A pinch of salt and black pepper
- 4 garlic cloves, minced

Directions:

1. In a ramekin, combine the shrimp with the cream cheese and the other ingredients, whisk, introduce in the oven and cook at 390 degrees F for 20 minutes.
2. Serve the dip warm.

Nutrition:

calories 200, fat 7, fiber 2, carbs 4, protein 6

Cheese Sticks

Prep time: 10 minutes | **Cooking time:** 12 minutes | **Servings:** 2

Ingredients:

- 1 egg, whisked
- A pinch of salt and black pepper
- 4 mozzarella cheese strings, halved
- 1 tablespoon Italian seasoning
- ½ cup olive oil
- 1 teaspoon rosemary, dried

Directions:

1. In a bowl, combine the egg with the seasoning and the other ingredients except the mozzarella strings and the oil and whisk.
2. Dip the mozzarella strips in the egg mixture.
3. Heat up a pan with the oil over medium high heat, add the cheese strings, cook them for 6 minutes on each side, arrange on a platter and serve.

Nutrition:

calories 140, fat 5, fiber 1, carbs 3, protein 4

Capers Salsa

Prep time: 10 minutes | **Servings:** 2

Ingredients:

- 2 avocados, peeled, pitted and cubed
- 1 tablespoon capers, drained
- 1 cup cherry tomatoes, cubed
- 1 tablespoon olive oil
- ½ teaspoon oregano, dried
- 1 tablespoon chives, chopped

Directions:

1. 1. In a bowl, combine the avocados with the tomatoes and the other ingredients, toss and serve as an appetizer.

Nutrition:

calories 100, fat 4, fiber 2, carbs 7, protein 7

Lamb and Garlic Dip

Prep time: 10 minutes | **Cooking time:** 25 minutes | **Servings:** 2

Ingredients:

- 1 pound lamb stew meat, ground
- 1 tablespoon olive oil
- 1 cup tomato passata (unsweetened)
- 2 garlic cloves, minced
- 1 tablespoon cilantro, chopped
- A pinch of salt and black pepper

Directions:

1. Heat up a pan with the oil over medium heat, add the garlic and the meat and brown for 5 minutes.
2. Add the rest of the ingredients, toss, cook for 20 minutes more, divide into bowls and serve as a party dip.

Nutrition:

calories 150, fat 4, fiber 0.4, carbs 1.1, protein 3

Mint Spread

Prep time: 10 minutes | **Servings:** 2

Ingredients:

- 2 avocados, peeled, pitted and mashed
- 1 cup coconut cream
- 1 tablespoon mint, chopped
- Juice of 1 lime
- A pinch of salt and black pepper
- 1 teaspoon chili powder

Directions:

1. 1. In a blender, combine the avocados with the cream and the other ingredients, pulse well, divide into bowls and serve.

Nutrition:

calories 140, fat 6, fiber 0, carbs 6, protein 15

Dijon Mustard Trout

Prep time: 5 minutes | **Cooking time:** 20 minutes | **Servings:** 2

Ingredients:
- 2 tablespoons olive oil
- 4 scallions, chopped
- 2 trout fillets, boneless
- 1 cup coconut cream
- A pinch of salt and black pepper
- 2 tablespoons Dijon mustard
- Juice of 1 lime

Directions:
1. Heat up a pan with the oil over medium heat, add the scallions and cook for 5 minutes.
2. Add the fish and the other ingredients, toss gently, cook over medium heat for 15 minutes more, divide between plates and serve.

Nutrition:
calories 171, fat 5, fiber 1, carbs 6, protein 23

Paprika Zucchini Chips

Prep time: 10 minutes | **Cooking time:** 20 minutes | **Servings:** 2

Ingredients:
- 2 zucchinis, thinly sliced
- 1 tablespoon olive oil
- 1 tablespoon lime juice
- A pinch of salt and black pepper
- 1 teaspoon sweet paprika

Directions:
1. Spread the zucchini slices on a baking sheet lined with parchment paper, add the oil and the other ingredients, toss and cook at 380 degrees F for 20 minutes.
2. Serve the chips as a snack.

Nutrition:
calories 95, fat 7.5, fiber 2.6, carbs 7.2, protein 2.5

Keto Salsa

Prep time: 10 minutes | **Servings:** 2

Ingredients:
- ½ cup black olives, pitted and chopped
- ½ cup kalamata olives, pitted and chopped
- A pinch of salt and black pepper
- 1 cup cherry tomatoes, halved
- 1 cucumber, sliced
- 1 tablespoon olive oil
- Juice of ½ lime
- 1 tablespoons chives, chopped

Directions:
1. 1. In a bowl, combine the olives with the tomatoes and the other ingredients, toss and serve.

Nutrition:
calories 177, fat 14.5, fiber 4, carbs 13.3, protein 2.4

Green Dip

Prep time: 5 minutes | **Cooking time:** 15 minutes | **Servings:** 2

Ingredients:
- 1 tablespoon olive oil
- 1 pound baby spinach
- 1 cup coconut cream
- 4 scallions, chopped
- A pinch of salt and black pepper
- ½ teaspoon coriander, ground
- ½ teaspoon rosemary, dried

Directions:
1. Heat up a pan with the oil over medium heat, add the scallions and cook for 2 minutes.
2. Add the spinach and the other ingredients, whisk, cook for 13 minutes more, blend using an immersion blender, divide into bowls and serve.

Nutrition:
calories 30, fat 3, fiber 1.2, carbs 0.5, protein 1

Basil Pesto Dip

Prep time: 10 minutes | **Servings:** 2

Ingredients:
- 1 cup black olives, pitted and cubed
- 1 cup green olives, pitted and cubed
- Salt and black pepper to the taste
- 2 tablespoons basil pesto
- 1 cup cream cheese
- 1 tablespoons basil, chopped

Directions:
1. 1. In a bowl, combine the olives with the pesto, cream cheese and the other ingredients, pulse well and serve as a party dip.

Nutrition:
calories 110, fat 10, fiber 0, carbs 1.4, protein 3

Coconut Cream Dip

Prep time: 10 minutes | **Servings:** 2

Ingredients:
- 2 teaspoons olive oil
- 1 cup mint, chopped
- 1 cup coconut cream
- 2 garlic cloves, minced
- ½ teaspoon cumin, ground
- 1 tablespoon almonds, chopped
- A pinch of salt and black pepper

Directions:
1. 1. In a blender, combine the mint with the cream and the other ingredients, pulse well and serve.

Nutrition:
calories 30, fat 3, fiber 1.2, carbs 0.5, protein 1

Cilantro Sea Bass

Prep time: 10 minutes | **Cooking time:** 20 minutes | **Servings:** 2

Ingredients:
- 2 sea bass fillets, boneless
- 1 tablespoon avocado oil
- A pinch of salt and black pepper
- 2 tablespoons cilantro, chopped
- 1 tablespoon lime juice

Directions:
1. Heat up a pan with the oil over medium heat, add the fish and cook it for 5 minutes on each side.
2. Add the lime juice and the other ingredients, toss, cook fro 10 minutes more, divide between plates and serve.

Nutrition:
calories 245, fat 12, fiber 1, carbs 3, protein 23

Scallions Shrimps

Prep time: 10 minutes | **Cooking time:** 10 minutes | **Servings:** 2

Ingredients:
- 1 pound shrimp, peeled and deveined
- 2 scallions, chopped
- 1 tablespoon parsley, chopped
- 2 tablespoons olive oil
- Juice of 1 lime
- A pinch of salt and black pepper

Directions:
1. Heat up a pan with the oil over medium heat, add the scallions and cook for 2 minutes.
2. Add the shrimp and the other ingredients, cook over medium heat for 6 minutes more, divide between plates and serve.

Nutrition:
calories 205, fat 9.1, fiber 0.6, carbs 4.1, protein 26.2

Sun Dried Tomatoes and Olives Salsa

Prep time: 0 minutes | **Servings:** 2

Ingredients:

- 1 cup sun-dried tomatoes, cubed
- 1 cup kalamata olives, pitted and halved
- 1 tablespoon balsamic vinegar
- A pinch of salt and black pepper
- ¼ cup pine nuts, toasted and chopped
- 1 tablespoon chives, chopped

Directions:

1. 1. In a bowl, combine the tomatoes with the olives and the other ingredients, toss and serve.

Nutrition:

calories 240, fat 12, fiber 3, carbs 5, protein 12

Avocado Dip

Prep time: 10 minutes | **Servings:** 4

Ingredients:

- 3 spring onions, chopped
- 2 avocados, pitted, peeled and chopped
- 3 jalapeno pepper, chopped
- A pinch of salt and black pepper
- 2 tablespoons cumin powder
- 2 tablespoons lime juice
- 1 tablespoon olive oil

Directions:

1. 1. In a blender, combine the avocados with the spring onions and the other ingredients, pulse well, divide into bowls and serve as a party dip.

Nutrition:

calories 120, fat 2, fiber 2, carbs 0.4, protein 4

Cumin Bowls

Prep time: 5 minutes | **Cooking time:** 20 minutes | **Servings:** 2

Ingredients:

- 2 cups radishes, halved
- 2 tablespoons parmesan, shredded
- 1 teaspoon cumin, ground
- 1 teaspoon rosemary dried
- 1 teaspoon sweet paprika
- 2 tablespoons olive oil
- A pinch of salt and black pepper

Directions:

1. In a roasting pan, combine the radishes with the parmesan and the other ingredients, toss and roast at 400 degrees F for 20 minutes.
2. Divide into bowls and serve as a snack.

Nutrition:

calories 120, fat 2, fiber 1, carbs 2, protein 7

Asparagus and Lime Zest Bowls

Prep time: 10 minutes | **Cooking time:** 20 minutes | **Servings:** 2

Ingredients:

- 1 cup asparagus, halved
- 1 and ½ teaspoons lime zest, grated
- 1 tablespoon lime juice
- 1 tablespoon olive oil
- ½ teaspoon sweet paprika

Directions:

1. In a roasting pan, combine the asparagus with the lime zest and the other ingredients, toss and cook at 390 degrees F for 20 minutes.
2. Divide into bowls and serve as a snack.

Nutrition:

calories 90, fat 1, fiber 1, carbs 0.6, protein 3

Garlic Wings

Prep time: 10 minutes | **Cooking time:** 20 minutes | **Servings:** 2

Ingredients:

- 1 pound chicken wings, cut in halves
- A pinch of salt and black pepper
- ½ teaspoon Italian seasoning
- 2 tablespoons olive oil
- 2 teaspoons red pepper flakes, crushed
- 1 teaspoon garlic powder

Directions:

1. In a bowl, combine the chicken wings with the seasoning and the other ingredients, toss well, spread them on a baking sheet lined with parchment paper and bake at 400 degrees F for 20 minutes.
2. Arrange the wings on a platter and serve.

Nutrition:

calories 134, fat 8, fiber 1, carbs 0.5, protein 14

Greens and Capers Salad

Prep time: 5 minutes | **Servings:** 2

Ingredients:

- 2 avocados, peeled, pitted and cubed
- 1 tablespoon capers, drained
- 1 cup cherry tomatoes, halved
- 1 cup baby spinach
- A pinch of salt and black pepper
- 2 green onions, chopped
- 1 tablespoon balsamic vinegar

Directions:

1. 1. In a bowl, combine the avocados with the capers, tomatoes and the other ingredients, toss and serve.

Nutrition:

calories 220, fat 7, fiber 2, carbs 6, protein 10

Chives Salsa

Prep time: 10 minutes | **Servings:** 2

Ingredients:

- 2 jalapenos, chopped
- 1 cup cherry tomatoes, halved
- 1 cup cucumber, cubed
- 1 tablespoon balsamic vinegar
- 1 tablespoon chives, chopped
- A pinch of salt and black pepper

Directions:

1. 1. In a bowl, combine the cherry tomatoes with the cucumber and the other ingredients, toss, and serve as an appetizer.

Nutrition:

calories 200, fat 16, fiber 1, carbs 1, protein 13

Cucumber and Dill Dip

Prep time: 10 minutes | **Servings:** 2

Ingredients:

- 2 tablespoons olive oil
- 2 cucumbers, cubed
- 1 cup cream cheese, soft
- 1 tablespoon dill, chopped
- A pinch of salt and black pepper
- Salt and black pepper to the taste

Directions:

1. 1. In a blender, combine the cucumbers with the oil and the other ingredients, pulse well, divide into bowls and serve.

Nutrition:

calories 50, fat 3, fiber 0.1, carbs 0.3, protein 2

Salmon Mix

Prep time: 10 minutes | **Servings:** 2

Ingredients:

- 1 pound smoked salmon fillets, cut into strips
- 1 tablespoon olive oil
- A pinch of salt and black pepper
- 1/3 cup cilantro, chopped
- 2 teaspoons lime juice
- 1 tablespoon lime zest, grated

Directions:

1. In a bowl combine the salmon with the oil, cilantro and the other ingredients, toss, arrange on a platter and serve.

Nutrition:

calories 30, fat 11, fiber 1, carbs 1, protein 2

Keto Eggs Salad

Prep time: 6 minutes | **Servings:** 2

Ingredients:

- 2 eggs, hard boiled, peeled and cubed
- ½ pound shrimp, peeled, deveined and cooked
- 1 tablespoon olive oil
- 2 scallions, chopped
- 1 cup baby arugula
- 1 tablespoon lime juice
- Salt and black pepper to the taste

Directions:

1. In a bowl, combine the eggs with the shrimp and the other ingredients, toss, divide into smaller bowls and serve.

Nutrition:

calories 122, fat 8, fiber 1, carbs 4, protein 7

Dijon Shrimp Skewers

Prep time: 10 minutes | **Cooking time:** 10 minutes | **Servings:** 2

Ingredients:

- 1 red bell pepper, cut in chunks
- 1 green bell pepper, cut into chunks
- 1 pound shrimp, peeled and deveined
- 4 garlic cloves, minced
- 1 tablespoon olive oil
- Salt and black pepper to the taste
- 2 tablespoons Dijon mustard
- ¼ cup lemon juice

Directions:

1. In a bowl, combine the peppers with the shrimp and the other ingredients and toss well.
2. Arrange the peppers and shrimp on skewers, place them on your preheated grill over medium high heat, cook for 5 minutes on each side, transfer to a platter and serve as an appetizer.

Nutrition:

calories 246, fat 12, fiber 1, carbs 4, protein 26

Keto Vegetables Rolls

Prep time: 10 minutes | **Servings:** 2

Ingredients:

- 2 cucumbers, thinly sliced lengthwise
- 2 tablespoons mint, chopped
- 1 cup cream cheese
- Salt and black pepper to the taste
- 1 tablespoon basil, chopped

Directions:

1. In a bowl, combine the cream cheese with the other ingredients except the cucumbers and stir well.
2. Arrange the cucumber slices on a working surface, divide the cheese mix, roll, arrange the rolls on a platter and serve.

Nutrition:

calories 40, fat 3, fiber 0.3, carbs 1, protein 2

Fennel Seeds Shrimp

Prep time: 10 minutes | **Cooking time:** 10 minutes | **Servings:** 2

Ingredients:

- 1 teaspoon coriander, ground
- ½ teaspoon mustard seeds, crushed
- ½ teaspoon fennel seeds, crushed
- 1 teaspoon sweet paprika
- 1 teaspoon garlic powder
- ¼ teaspoon nutmeg, ground
- A pinch of salt and black pepper
- 1 pound shrimp, peeled and deveined
- 4 scallions, chopped
- Juice of ½ lime
- 1 tablespoon olive oil
- ½ cup chicken broth
- 1 tablespoon ghee, melted

Directions:

1. Heat up a pan with the ghee and the oil over medium heat, add the scallions and cook for 4 minutes stirring often.
2. Add the shrimp and the other ingredients, toss, cook for 6 minutes more, divide into bowls and serve.

Nutrition:

calories 200, fat 5, fiber 7, carbs 4, protein 20

Parsley and Shrimps Bowl

Prep time: 10 minutes | **Cooking time:** 15 minutes | **Servings:** 2

Ingredients:

- 1 tablespoon olive oil
- 1 pound shrimp, peeled and deveined
- A pinch of salt and black pepper
- ½ pound Brussels sprouts, trimmed and halved
- 1 tablespoon parsley, chopped
- 1 tablespoon lemon juice
- 1 tablespoon lemon zest, grated
- ½ cup chicken broth
- ½ teaspoon sweet paprika

Directions:

1. Heat up a pan with the oil over medium heat, add the sprouts and cook for 5 minutes.
2. Add the shrimp and the other ingredients, toss, cook for 10 minutes more, divide between plates and serve.

Nutrition:

calories 200, fat 11, fiber 2, carbs 1, protein 13

Ginger Tuna

Prep time: 10 minutes | **Cooking time:** 15 minutes | **Servings:** 2

Ingredients:

- 1 pound tuna fillets, boneless, skinless and cubed
- 1 tablespoon olive oil
- Zest of 1 lime, grated
- Juice of 1 lime
- 1 teaspoon chili powder
- 1 teaspoon cumin, ground
- 1 Serrano chili pepper, chopped
- ½ teaspoon ginger, grated
- A pinch of salt and black pepper
- ¼ cup cilantro, chopped
- ¼ cup scallions, chopped

Directions:

1. Heat up a pan with the oil over medium heat, add the scallions, ginger and the other ingredients except the tuna and cook for 5 minutes.
2. Add the tuna, toss gently, cook for 10 minutes more, divide between plates and serve.

Nutrition:

calories 100, fat 1, fiber 0, carbs 2, protein 5

Scallions Dip

Prep time: 10 minutes | **Cooking time:** 30 minutes | **Servings:** 2

Ingredients:
- ½ pound pork stew meat, ground
- 3 scallions, chopped
- 1 tablespoon avocado oil
- 1 cup tomato passata (unsweetened)
- A pinch of salt and black pepper
- ¼ cup green onions, chopped

Directions:
1. Heat up a pan with the oil over medium heat, add the scallions and green onions and cook for 5 minutes.
2. Add the meat and brown for 5 minutes more.
3. Add the rest of the ingredients, toss, cook for 20 minutes, divide into bowls and serve as a party dip.

Nutrition:
calories 261, fat 11.9, fiber 1.2, carbs 3, protein 33.9

Balsamic Tuna with Spring Onions

Prep time: 5 minutes | **Cooking time:** 15 minutes | **Servings:** 2

Ingredients:
- 2 tablespoons olive oil
- 3 spring onions, chopped
- 1 pound tuna fillets, boneless and cubed
- 3 tablespoon balsamic vinegar
- 2 tablespoons mint, chopped
- 1 tablespoon pine nuts, chopped
- Juice of 1 lime
- 1 jalapeno pepper, chopped
- A pinch of salt and black pepper
- 1 teaspoon red pepper flakes, crushed

Directions:
1. In a blender, combine half of the oil with the spring onions and the other ingredients except the tuna and pulse well.
2. Heat up a pan with the rest of the oil over medium heat, add the tuna and cook for 3 minutes on each side.
3. Add the mint sauce, toss gently, cook for 9 minutes more, divide between plates and serve.

Nutrition:
calories 186, fat 3, fiber 1, carbs 4, protein 20

Nutmeg Salmon Bowl

Prep time: 5 minutes | **Cooking time:** 15 minutes | **Servings:** 2

Ingredients:
- 2 salmon fillets, boneless and cubed
- 1 tablespoon walnuts, chopped
- 1 tablespoon avocado oil
- ½ teaspoon sweet paprika
- ½ teaspoon turmeric powder
- ¼ cup chicken broth
- A pinch of salt and black pepper
- 3 green onions, chopped
- ¼ teaspoon nutmeg, ground
- 1 tablespoon chives, chopped

Directions:
1. Heat up a pan with the oil over medium high heat, add the green onions, paprika and turmeric and cook for 2 minutes.
2. Add the fish, walnuts and the other ingredients, toss, cook for 13 minutes more, divide into bowls and serve.

Nutrition:
calories 430, fat 30, fiber 3, carbs 7, protein 50

Garlic Powder Dip

Prep time: 5 minutes | **Servings:** 2

Ingredients:
- 1 cup coconut cream
- 2 tablespoons pine nuts, toasted
- 1 tablespoon avocado oil
- 2 red chilies, minced
- ¼ teaspoon garlic powder
- A pinch of salt and black pepper
- 1 tablespoon chives, chopped

Directions:
1. 1. In a blender, combine the cream with the pine nuts, oil and the other ingredients, pulse well, divide into bowls and serve.

Nutrition:
calories 130, fat 3.8, fiber 1, carbs 2.2, protein 5

Spring Onions Dip

Prep time: 10 minutes | **Cooking time:** 20 minutes | **Servings:** 2

Ingredients:
- 1 cup coconut cream
- 1 tablespoon ghee, melted
- 1 cup coconut, unsweetened and shredded
- 2 spring onions, chopped
- ½ teaspoon chives, chopped
- ½ teaspoon chili powder
- A pinch of salt and black pepper

Directions:
1. Heat up a pan with the ghee over medium heat, add the onions and cook for 5 minutes.
2. Add the cream and the other ingredients, whisk, cook for 15 minutes more, divide into bowls and serve.

Nutrition:
calories 481, fat 48.5, fiber 6.9, carbs 14.2, protein 4.5

Vegetable Spread

Prep time: 5 minutes | **Cooking time:** 20 minutes | **Servings:** 2

Ingredients:
- 2 cups cauliflower florets
- 1 cup coconut cream
- 1 tablespoon sesame seed paste
- 1 tablespoon olive oil
- 2 garlic clove, minced
- A pinch of cayenne pepper

Directions:
1. Heat up a pan with the oil over medium heat, add the garlic and cook for 2 minutes.
2. Add the cauliflower and the other ingredients, whisk, cook for 18 minutes more, blend using an immersion blender, divide into bowls and serve.

Nutrition:
calories 392, fat 38, fiber 5.8, carbs 14.1, protein 5.7

Coconut Muffins

Prep time: 10 minutes | **Cooking time:** 24 minutes | **Servings:** 2

Ingredients:
- 1 cup coconut flour
- 2 cups spinach, torn
- A pinch of salt and black pepper
- 2 eggs, whisked
- 2 tablespoons ghee, melted
- 1 teaspoon baking powder
- A pinch of salt and black pepper

Directions:
1. In a bowl, combine the spinach with the flour and the other ingredients, whisk well and divide into a muffin tray.
2. Introduce in the oven at 350 degrees F, bake for 24 minutes and serve cold as a snack.

Nutrition:
calories 247, fat 22.3, fiber 2.2, carbs 6.2, protein 6.6

Cheese Dip

Prep time: 10 minutes | **Cooking time:** 20 minutes | **Servings:** 2

Ingredients:

- 1 cup cheddar cheese, shredded
- 1 cup coconut cream
- 2 tablespoons parmesan, grated
- 4 scallions, chopped
- 1 tablespoon ghee, melted
- A pinch of salt and black pepper
- 1 tablespoon chives, chopped
- 1 teaspoon turmeric powder

Directions:

1. In a ramekin, combine the cheese with the scallions and the other ingredients, whisk, introduce in the oven and cook at 380 degrees F for 20 minutes.
2. Serve the dip right away.

Nutrition:

calories 200, fat 5.4, fiber 4, carbs 5.4, protein 5.5

Chicken Muffins

Prep time: 10 minutes | **Cooking time:** 30 minutes | **Servings:** 2

Ingredients:

- ½ cup coconut flour
- ½ pound chicken meat, ground
- 1 egg, whisked
- A pinch of salt and black pepper
- 2 spring onions, chopped
- A drizzle of olive oil
- ¼ teaspoon baking powder
- ¼ cup coconut milk

Directions:

1. In a bowl, combine the meat with the flour and the other ingredients except the oil and stir well.
2. Grease a muffin tray with the oil, divide the mix in each muffin mould, introduce in the oven at 360 degrees F and bake for 30 minutes.
3. Serve as an appetizer right away.

Nutrition:

calories 227, fat 9.7, fiber 4.4, carbs 7.8, protein 6.4

Seafood Meatballs

Prep time: 5 minutes | **Cooking time:** 6 minutes | **Servings:** 2

Ingredients:

- 1 pound shrimp, peeled, deveined, cooked and chopped
- 1 egg, whisked
- A pinch of salt and black pepper
- ¼ cup almond flour
- 2 tablespoons shallots, chopped
- 1 tablespoon chives, chopped
- ½ cup mozzarella cheese, shredded
- 2 tablespoons olive oil

Directions:

1. In a bowl, combine the shrimp with the egg, salt, pepper and the other ingredients except the oil, stir well and shape medium meatballs out of this mix.
2. Heat up a pan with the oil over medium high heat, add the meatballs, cook for 3 minutes on each side, arrange on a platter and serve.

Nutrition:

calories 80, fat 6, fiber 3, carbs 5, protein 7

Fish Platter

Prep time: 10 minutes | **Cooking time:** 12 minutes | **Servings:** 2

Ingredients:

- 2 tablespoons ghee, melted
- ½ pound salmon fillets, boneless and cubed
- 1 tablespoon balsamic vinegar
- 1 tablespoon chives, chopped
- A pinch of salt and black pepper

Directions:

1. 1. Heat up a pan with the ghee over medium heat, add the salmon bites and the other ingredients, toss gently, cook for 12 minutes, arrange on a platter and serve.

Nutrition:

calories 60, fat 5, fiber 1, carbs 0.7, protein 2

Kale and Parsley Dip

Prep time: 10 minutes | **Cooking time:** 25 minutes | **Servings:** 2

Ingredients:

- 1 cup kale
- ½ cup parmesan, grated
- ½ cup coconut cream
- ½ cup cream cheese, soft
- 1 tablespoon parsley, chopped
- 1 tablespoon lemon juice
- A pinch of salt and black pepper

Directions:

1. In a blender, combine the kale with the cream and the other ingredients, pulse, transfer to 2 ramekins, introduce in the oven and cook at 380 degrees F for 25 minutes.
2. Serve as a party dip.

Nutrition:

calories 345, fat 12, fiber 3, carbs 6, protein 11

Shrimp and Curry Powder Salsa

Prep time: 10 minutes | **Cooking time:** 10 minutes | **Servings:** 2

Ingredients:

- ½ pound shrimp, peeled and deveined
- 1 teaspoon garlic powder
- 2 spring onions, chopped
- ½ cup cherry tomatoes, cubed
- ½ cup black olives, pitted and cubed
- A pinch of salt and black pepper
- 1 tablespoon olive oil
- 1 teaspoon curry powder

Directions:

1. Heat up a pan with the oil over medium heat, add spring onions, curry and garlic powder, stir and cook for 2 minutes.
2. Add the shrimp and the other ingredients, toss, cook for 8 minutes more, divide into bowls and serve as an appetizer.

Nutrition:

calories 244, fat 20, fiber 3, carbs 7, protein 14

Italian Style Shrimps

Prep time: 5 minutes | **Cooking time:** 10 minutes | **Servings:** 2

Ingredients:

- 2 tablespoons basil pesto
- ½ pound shrimp, peeled and deveined
- 1 tablespoon olive oil
- Juice of 1 lime
- 2 tablespoons Italian seasoning
- A pinch of salt and black pepper

Directions:

1. 1. Heat up a pan with the oil over medium heat, add the shrimp and the other ingredients, toss, cook for 10 minutes, arrange on a platter and serve as an appetizer.

Nutrition:

calories 245, fat 12, fiber 5, carbs 3, protein 11

Basil Tuna and Cayenne Pepper Bowl

Prep time: 4 minutes | **Cooking time:** 14 minutes | **Servings:** 2

Ingredients:

- 1 pound tuna fillets, boneless and cubed
- 3 garlic cloves, minced
- 1 tablespoon olive oil
- 1 red bell pepper, chopped
- 1 zucchini, cubed
- 1 tablespoon basil, chopped
- 2 scallions, chopped
- ½ teaspoon sweet paprika
- ½ teaspoon garam masala
- A pinch of salt and black pepper
- A pinch of cayenne pepper
- 1 tablespoons cilantro, chopped

Directions:

1. Heat up a pan with the oil medium heat, add the garlic, pepper, zucchini and scallions, stir and cook for 4 minutes.
2. Add the tuna and the rest of the ingredients, toss, cook for 10 minutes more, divide between plates and serve.

Nutrition:

calories 345, fat 32, fiber 3, carbs 3, protein 13

Turmeric Calamari

Prep time: 10 minutes | **Cooking time:** 20 minutes | **Servings:** 2

Ingredients:

- 1 pound calamari, cut in medium rings
- 1 tablespoon avocado oil
- 2 scallions, chopped
- 1 cup cherry tomatoes, halved
- Juice of ½ lemon
- Zest of ½ lemon, grated
- A pinch of salt and black pepper
- ½ teaspoon turmeric powder

Directions:

1. Heat up a pan with the oil over medium heat, add the scallions and turmeric, stir and cook for 2 minutes.
2. Add calamari rings and the other ingredients, toss, cook for 18 minutes more, divide everything into bowls and serve.

Nutrition:

calories 368, fat 23, fiber 3, carbs 10, protein 34

Calamari with Zucchini Zoodles

Prep time: 10 minutes | **Cooking time:** 20 minutes | **Servings:** 2

Ingredients:

- 1 pound calamari rings
- 2 zucchinis, cut with a spiralizer
- 2 scallions, chopped
- 2 cherry tomatoes, cubed
- 1 tablespoon olive oil
- Juice of 1 lime
- A pinch of salt and black pepper
- 1 teaspoon chili powder
- ½ teaspoon oregano, dried
- 1 tablespoon parsley, chopped

Directions:

1. Heat up a pan with the oil over medium heat, add the scallions, chili powder and oregano, stir and cook for 2 minutes.
2. Add the calamari, stir and cook for 13 minutes more.
3. Add the rest of the ingredients, toss, cook for 5 minutes, divide into bowls and serve.

Nutrition:

calories 140, fat 10, fiber 3, carbs 6, protein 23

Shrimps with Fresh Fennel Bulb

Prep time: 5 minutes | **Cooking time:** 8 minutes | **Servings:** 2

Ingredients:

- 1 pound shrimp, peeled and deveined
- 1 tablespoon avocado oil
- 1 fennel bulb, sliced
- 1 teaspoon coriander, ground
- ½ teaspoon cumin, ground
- ½ teaspoon turmeric powder
- A pinch of salt and black pepper
- 2 tablespoons lime juice
- 2 tablespoons chives, chopped

Directions:

1. Heat up a pan with the oil over medium heat, add the fennel, coriander, cumin and turmeric and cook for 2 minutes.
2. Add the shrimp and the rest of the ingredients, cook over medium heat for 6 minutes more, divide into bowls and serve.

Nutrition:

calories 130, fat 2, fiber 3, carbs 1, protein 6

Shrimps with Endives

Prep time: 5 minutes | **Cooking time:** 10 minutes | **Servings:** 2

Ingredients:

- 1 pound shrimp, peeled and deveined
- 1 cup green beans, trimmed and halved
- 2 endives, trimmed and shredded
- 2 garlic cloves, minced
- ¼ cup chicken broth
- 2 tablespoons olive oil
- A pinch of salt and black pepper
- 1 teaspoon allspice
- 1 tablespoon chives, chopped

Directions:

1. Heat up a pan with the oil over medium heat, add the endives, garlic and allspice, stir and cook for 2 minutes.
2. Add the shrimp and the other ingredients, cook over medium heat for 8 minutes more, divide into bowls and serve.

Nutrition:

calories 120, fat 3, fiber 1, carbs 2, protein 6

Baby Spinach and Fish Salad

Prep time: 10 minutes | **Cooking time:** 14 minutes | **Servings:** 2

Ingredients:

- 1 pound tuna fillets, boneless and cubed
- 1 tablespoon olive oil
- 1 cup cherry tomatoes, halved
- ½ cup black olives, pitted and halved
- 1 cup baby spinach
- 1 tablespoon lime juice
- A pinch of salt and black pepper
- 1 tablespoon balsamic vinegar
- 1 tablespoon parsley, chopped
- ½ teaspoon red chili flakes

Directions:

1. Heat up a pan with the oil over medium heat and the tuna and cook for 5 minutes.
2. Add the tomatoes, olives and the other ingredients, toss gently and cook for 9 minutes more.
3. Divide the salad into bowls and serve warm.

Nutrition:

calories 240, fat 4, fiber 2, carbs 6, protein 9

Pesto Snack

Prep time: 10 minutes | **Cooking time:** 20 minutes | **Servings:** 2

Ingredients:

- 3 tablespoons basil pesto
- ½ teaspoon baking soda
- Salt and black pepper to the taste
- 1 cup coconut flour
- ¼ teaspoon basil, dried
- 1 garlic clove, minced
- A pinch of cayenne pepper
- 3 tablespoons ghee, melted

Directions:

1. In a bowl, combine the pesto with the coconut flour and the other ingredients, and stir well until your obtain a dough.
2. Spread this dough on a lined baking sheet, introduce in the oven at 325 degrees F and bake for 20 minutes.
3. Leave aside to cool down, cut the crackers and serve as a snack.

Nutrition:

calories 200, fat 20, fiber 1, carbs 4, protein 7

Curry and Garlic Shrimps

Prep time: 10 minutes | **Cooking time:** 15 minutes | **Servings:** 2

Ingredients:

- ½ pound shrimp, peeled and deveined
- 2 tablespoons ghee, melted
- 2 garlic cloves, minced
- ½ teaspoon curry powder
- 2 shallots, chopped
- A pinch of salt and black pepper
- 1 teaspoon turmeric powder
- 1 cup coconut cream
- ¼ cup cilantro, chopped

Directions:

1. Heat up a pot with the oil over medium heat, add the shallots, garlic and curry powder and cook for 2 minutes.
2. Add the shrimp and the remaining ingredients, cook over medium heat for 13 minutes, divide the mix into bowls and serve.

Nutrition:

calories 500, fat 34, fiber 4.1, carbs 6, protein 7.3

Cod with Coriander Sauce

Prep time: 10 minutes | **Cooking time:** 15 minutes | **Servings:** 2

Ingredients:

- 1 tablespoon ghee, melted
- 3 shallots, minced
- 2 garlic cloves, minced
- 2 cod fillets, boneless
- ½ teaspoon turmeric powder
- ½ teaspoon coriander, ground
- 1 tablespoon oregano, chopped
- 1 cup chicken broth
- A pinch of salt and black pepper

Directions:

1. Heat up a pan with the oil over medium heat, add the shallots, garlic, and oregano, stir and cook for 5 minutes.
2. Add the fish and the other ingredients, toss gently, cook over medium heat for 10 minutes more, divide between plates and serve.

Nutrition:

calories 250, fat 12, fiber 3, carbs 5, protein 20

Sour Cumin Shrimp

Prep time: 5 minutes | **Cooking time:** 10 minutes | **Servings:** 2

Ingredients:

- 1 pound shrimp, peeled and deveined
- Juice of 1 lime
- 1 cup chicken broth
- 2 shallots, chopped
- 2 garlic cloves, minced
- ½ teaspoon cumin, ground
- A pinch of salt and black pepper
- 1 tablespoon parsley, chopped

Directions:

1. Heat up a pan with the oil over medium high heat, add the shallots, garlic and the cumin and sauté for 2 minutes.
2. Add the shrimp and the other ingredients, toss, and cook for 8 minutes more.
3. Divide everything between plates and serve.

Nutrition:

calories 149, fat 1, fiber 3, carbs 1, protein 6

Chia and Flaxseeds Muffins

Prep time: 10 minutes | **Cooking time:** 20 minutes | **Servings:** 2

Ingredients:

- 3 tablespoons walnuts, chopped
- ¼ cup chia seeds
- ¾ cup coconut cream
- 2 tablespoons flaxseed meal
- ¼ cup coconut flour
- ½ teaspoon nutmeg, ground
- ½ teaspoon baking soda
- 1 egg, whisked
- ½ teaspoon baking powder
- A pinch of salt

Directions:

1. In a bowl, combine the seeds with the chia seeds and the other ingredients, whisk well and divide into a muffin tray.
2. Introduce in the oven at 350 degrees F and bake for 20 minutes.
3. Leave the muffins to cool down and serve them as a snack.

Nutrition:

calories 50, fat 3, fiber 1, carbs 2, protein 2

Avocado Mix with Calamari Rings

Prep time: 10 minutes | **Cooking time:** 20 minutes | **Servings:** 2

Ingredients:

- 1 pound calamari rings
- ½ cup chicken broth
- 1 tablespoon olive oil
- 1 tablespoon ghee, melted
- 2 small avocados, pitted, peeled and chopped
- 1 green chili, minced
- Juice of 1 lime
- Zest of 1 lime, grated
- A pinch of salt and black pepper
- 2 spring onions, chopped

Directions:

1. In a blender, combine the oil with the avocado, chili, lime juice, zest, salt, pepper and spring onions and pulse well.
2. Heat up a pan with the ghee over medium heat, add the calamari and cook for 5 minutes.
3. Add the stock and guacamole mix, toss, cook for 15 minutes more, divide into bowls and serve.

Nutrition:

calories 500, fat 43, fiber 6, carbs 7, protein 20

Red Pepper Flakes Trout

Prep time: 10 minutes | **Cooking time:** 12 minutes | **Servings:** 2

Ingredients:

- 2 trout fillets, boneless
- 1 tablespoon ghee, melted
- 1 tablespoon oregano, chopped
- 1 teaspoon red pepper flakes, crushed
- 1 teaspoon parsley, chopped
- 2 garlic cloves, minced
- Juice of 1 lime
- A pinch of salt and black pepper

Directions:

1. Heat up a pan with the ghee over medium heat, add the garlic and cook for 2 minutes.
2. Add trout fillets and the other ingredients, cook them for 5 minutes on each side, divide everything between plates and serve.

Nutrition:

calories 224, fat 15, fiber 2, carbs 3, protein 4

Cauli and Shrimps

Prep time: 10 minutes | **Cooking time:** 10 minutes | **Servings:** 2

Ingredients:

- 1 pound shrimp, peeled and deveined
- 1 cup cauliflower florets
- 1 avocado, peeled, pitted and cubed
- 1 tablespoon balsamic vinegar
- 1 tablespoon olive oil
- 1/3 cup cilantro, chopped
- A pinch of salt and black pepper
- ½ teaspoon cumin, ground
- ½ teaspoon sweet paprika

Directions:

1. 1. Heat up a pan with the oil over medium heat, add the shrimp, cauliflower and the other ingredients, toss, cook for 10 minutes, divide into bowls and serve.

Nutrition:

calories 160, fat 3, fiber 2, carbs 1, protein 8

Shrimps in Sauce

Prep time: 5 minutes | **Cooking time:** 10 minutes | **Servings:** 2

Ingredients:

- 1 pound shrimp, peeled and deveined
- A pinch of salt and black pepper
- 1 tablespoon olive oil
- 2 red chilies, minced
- 1 teaspoon hot paprika
- ½ cup chicken broth
- 1 tablespoon chives, chopped
- 1 tablespoon balsamic vinegar

Directions:

1. In a blender, combine the chilies with the stock, paprika and vinegar and pulse well.
2. Heat up a pan with the oil over medium heat, add the shrimp and the sauce, toss and cook for 10 minutes.
3. Divide between plates and serve.

Nutrition:

calories 50, fat 2, fiber 0, carbs 4, protein 2

Shrimps with Green Beans

Prep time: 10 minutes | **Cooking time:** 12 minutes | **Servings:** 2

Ingredients:

- 2 garlic cloves, minced
- 2 scallions, chopped
- 1 cucumber, cubed
- 1 cup green beans trimmed and halved
- 1 pound shrimp, peeled and deveined
- 2 tablespoons olive oil
- 1 tablespoon balsamic vinegar
- A pinch of salt and black pepper
- 1 tablespoon parsley, chopped

Directions:

1. Heat up a pan with the oil over medium heat, add the scallions and the garlic and cook for 2 minutes.
2. Add the shrimp and the other ingredients, toss, cook for 10 minutes more, divide the mix into bowls and serve.

Nutrition:

calories 240, fat 12, fiber 6.1, carbs 5.6, protein 25

Chili Cod

Prep time: 10 minutes | **Cooking time:** 20 minutes | **Servings:** 2

Ingredients:

- 2 cod fillets, boneless
- 1 tablespoons olive oil
- 1 cup cherry tomatoes, halved
- 2 shallots, chopped
- ½ cup chicken broth
- ½ teaspoon chili powder
- A pinch of salt and black pepper
- 1 tablespoon chives, chopped

Directions:

1. Heat up a pan with the oil over medium heat, add the shallots and cook for 5 minutes.
2. Add the fish and the rest of the ingredients, toss gently, cook for 15 minutes more, divide between plates and serve.

Nutrition:

calories 200, fat 6, fiber 1, carbs 4, protein 20

Shrimps with Almonds and Parmesan

Prep time: 10 minutes | **Cooking time:** 10 minutes | **Servings:** 2

Ingredients:

- 1 pound shrimp, peeled and deveined
- 1 tablespoon olive oil
- Juice of 1 lime
- 2 scallions, chopped
- 1 tablespoon almonds, chopped
- 2 tablespoons parmesan, grated
- 1 teaspoon coriander, ground
- 1 tablespoon chives, chopped
- A pinch of salt and black pepper

Directions:

1. Heat up a pan with the oil over medium heat, add the scallions and almonds and cook for 2 minutes.
2. Add the shrimp and the other ingredients, toss, cook for 8 minutes more, divide between plates and serve.

Nutrition:

calories 185, fat 11, fiber 0, carbs 2, protein 13

Rosemary Sea Bass

Prep time: 10 minutes | **Cooking time:** 20 minutes | **Servings:** 2

Ingredients:

- 1 pound sea bass fillets, boneless and cubed
- 1 avocado, peeled, pitted and cubed
- 2 tablespoons green onions, chopped
- 2 tablespoons olive oil
- 1 teaspoon rosemary, dried
- 1 teaspoon cumin, ground
- 1 tablespoon chives, chopped

Directions:

1. Heat up a pan with the oil over medium heat, add the green onions and cook for 2 minutes.
2. Add the fish and the other ingredients, cook over medium heat for 18 minutes more, divide into bowls and serve.

Nutrition:

calories 144, fat 12, fiber 2, carbs 5, protein 5

Trout Bowl

Prep time: 10 minutes | **Cooking time:** 20 minutes | **Servings:** 2

Ingredients:

- 1 pound trout fillets, boneless
- 2 endives, shredded
- 2 tablespoons ghee, melted
- Zest of 1 lime, grated
- Juice of 1 lime
- ½ cup chicken broth
- 1 teaspoon sweet paprika
- ½ teaspoon chili powder
- A pinch of salt and black pepper
- 1 tablespoon chives, chopped

Directions:

1. In a roasting pan, combine the trout fillets with the endives, ghee and the other ingredients, toss and cook at 390 degrees F for 20 minutes.
2. Divide the mix between plates and serve.

Nutrition:

calories 400, fat 24, fiber 4, carbs 12, protein 25

Oregano and Chili Cod

Prep time: 10 minutes | **Cooking time:** 12 minutes | **Servings:** 2

Ingredients:

- 2 cod fillets, boneless
- 1 tablespoon avocado oil
- 3 garlic cloves, minced
- A pinch of salt and black pepper
- 1 teaspoon chili powder
- 1 teaspoon coriander, ground
- 1 tablespoon oregano, chopped
- ½ teaspoon chili pepper, crushed

Directions:

1. Heat up a pan with the oil over medium high heat, add the garlic and chili pepper and cook for 2 minutes.
2. Add the fish and the other ingredients, cook for 10 minutes, divide between plates and serve.

Nutrition:

calories 154, fat 3, fiber 0.5, carbs 4, protein 24

Artichoke and Parmesan Spread

Prep time: 10 minutes | **Cooking time:** 20 minutes | **Servings:** 2

Ingredients:

- 1 cup cream cheese, soft
- 1 cup artichoke hearts, chopped
- ¼ cup shallot, chopped
- 1 tablespoon olive oil
- 2 garlic cloves, minced
- ½ cup parmesan cheese, grated
- 1 tablespoon balsamic vinegar
- A pinch of salt and black pepper
- cup baby spinach

Directions:

1. In a bowl, combine the artichokes with the cream cheese and the other ingredients, whisk, transfer to 2 ramekins, and bake at 380 degrees F for 20 minutes.
2. Serve the spread right away.

Nutrition:

calories 144, fat 12, fiber 2, carbs 5, protein 5

Rosemary and Chives Salmon

Prep time: 10 minutes | **Cooking time:** 12 minutes | **Servings:** 2

Ingredients:

- 1 pound salmon fillets, boneless and cubed
- 1 tablespoon olive oil
- 1 cucumber, cubed
- ½ teaspoon chili powder
- ½ teaspoon rosemary, dried
- 1 tablespoons lemon juice
- A pinch of salt and black pepper
- 1 tablespoon chives, chopped

Directions:

1. Heat up a pan with the oil over medium heat, add the salmon and chili powder and cook for 4 minutes.
2. Add the cucumber and the other ingredients, toss gently, cook for 8 minutes more, divide between plates and serve.

Nutrition:

calories 200, fat 20, fiber 1, carbs 0, protein 20

Coriander Calamari with Olives

Prep time: 10 minutes | **Cooking time:** 20 minutes | **Servings:** 2

Ingredients:

- 1 pound calamari rings
- 1 cup black olives, pitted and halved
- 1 tablespoon olive oil
- 1 teaspoon coriander, ground
- ½ teaspoon sweet paprika
- 1 tablespoon ghee, melted
- 3 garlic cloves, minced
- A pinch of salt and black pepper
- Juice of ½ lemon
- 1 tablespoon cilantro, chopped

Directions:

1. Heat up a patn with the oil and the ghee over medium heat, add the garlic and calamari and cook for 5 minutes.
2. Add the rest of the ingredients, toss, cook for 15 minutes more, divide into bowls and serve.

Nutrition:

calories 100, fat 2, fiber 1, carbs 1, protein 20

Green Onions Calamari

Prep time: 10 minutes | **Cooking time:** 20 minutes | **Servings:** 2

Ingredients:

- 3 scallions, chopped
- 1 pound calamari rings
- 2 garlic cloves, minced
- 3 green onions, chopped
- 1 tablespoon avocado oil
- 1 tablespoon balsamic vinegar
- Salt and black pepper to the taste
- Juice of 1 lime
- 1 tablespoon chives, chopped

Directions:

1. Heat up a pan with the oil over medium heat, add the scallions, garlic and green onions and sauté for 2 minutes.
2. Add calamari and the other ingredients, toss, cook for 18 minutes more, divide into bowls and serve.

Nutrition:

calories 200, fat 4, fiber 2, carbs 2, protein 7

Aromatic Shrimps with Pine Nuts

Prep time: 10 minutes | **Cooking time:** 10 minutes | **Servings:** 2

Ingredients:

- 1 pound shrimp, peeled and deveined
- 1 tablespoon olive oil
- 1 tablespoon lime juice
- 1 tablespoon pine nuts, toasted
- ½ teaspoon chili powder
- ½ teaspoon sweet paprika
- ½ teaspoon oregano, dried
- A pinch of salt and black pepper

Directions:

1. 1. Heat up a pan with the oil over medium heat, add the shrimp, lime juice and the other ingredients, toss, cook for 10 minutes, divide into bowls and serve.

Nutrition:

calories 70, fat 2, fiber 0, carbs 1, protein 1

Coconut Milk Cod

Prep time: 5 minutes | **Cooking time:** 15 minutes | **Servings:** 2

Ingredients:

- 1 tablespoon ghee, melted
- 1 pound cod fillets, boneless and cubed
- 1 cup broccoli florets
- ¼ cup coconut milk
- A pinch of salt and black pepper
- 2 garlic cloves, minced
- ¼ cup chicken broth
- 1 tablespoon chives, chopped

Directions:

1. Heat up a pan with the ghee over medium heat, add the garlic and cook for 2 minutes.
2. Add the fish and cook it for 5 minutes more.
3. Add the broccoli and the other ingredients, toss, cook for 8 minutes, divide into bowls and serve.

Nutrition:

calories 245, fat 7, fiber 4, carbs 6, protein 20

Coriander Cod

Prep time: 10 minutes | **Cooking time:** 20 minutes | **Servings:** 2

Ingredients:

- 3 scallions, chopped
- 2 garlic cloves, minced
- 1 cup coconut cream
- 1 tablespoon basil, chopped
- 2 tablespoons olive oil
- ½ teaspoon coriander, ground
- 2 cod fillets, boneless
- A pinch of salt and black pepper

Directions:

1. Heat up a pan with the oil over medium heat, add the scallions and the garlic and cook for 5 minutes.
2. Add fish, basil and the other ingredients, toss gently, cook for 15 minutes more, divide everything between plates and serve.

Nutrition:

calories 230, fat 12, fiber 1, carbs 4, protein 9

Avocado with Cod

Prep time: 10 minutes | **Cooking time:** 14 minutes | **Servings:** 2

Ingredients:

- 2 cod fillets, boneless
- 1 tablespoon olive oil
- 2 avocados, peeled, pitted and cubed
- 1 cup cherry tomatoes, halved
- 1 tablespoon lime juice
- ½ cup chicken broth
- A pinch of salt and black pepper
- 1 tablespoon chives, chopped

Directions:

1. Heat up a pan with the oil over medium heat, add the fish and cook for 2 minutes on each side.
2. Add the rest of the ingredients, toss gently, cook for 10 minutes more, divide between plates and serve.

Nutrition:

calories 150, fat 4, fiber 2, carbs 1, protein 10

Tuna with Vegetables

Prep time: 5 minutes | **Cooking time:** 14 minutes | **Servings:** 2

Ingredients:

- ½ pound tuna fillets, boneless, skinless and cubed
- 1 tablespoon olive oil
- 1 zucchini, cubed
- 2 scallions, chopped
- 1 tablespoon lime juice
- 1 tablespoon chives, chopped
- A pinch of salt and black pepper

Directions:

1. Heat up a pan the oil over medium high heat, add the scallions and the zucchini and cook for 4 minutes.
2. Add the fish and the other ingredients, toss gently, cook for 10 more minutes, divide into bowls and serve.

Nutrition:

calories 447, fat 38.7, fiber 10.3, carbs 1.1, protein 24.1

Tender Salmon with Ghee

Prep time: 10 minutes | **Cooking time:** 14 minutes | **Servings:** 2

Ingredients:

- 2 salmon fillets, boneless
- 1 tablespoon ghee, melted
- 1 teaspoon chili powder
- 2 green chilies, minced
- 1 cup tomato passata (unsweetened)
- A pinch of salt and black pepper
- 1 teaspoon cumin, ground

Directions:

1. Heat up a pan with the ghee over medium-high heat, add the chilies and the chili powder and cook for 4 minutes.
2. Add the fish and the rest of the ingredients, toss, cook for 10 minutes more, divide between plates and serve.

Nutrition:

calories 300, fat 14, fiber 4, carbs 5, protein 20

Tender Sour Tuna

Prep time: 5 minutes | **Cooking time:** 14 minutes | **Servings:** 2

Ingredients:

- 1 pound tuna fillets, boneless and cubed
- 1 tablespoon avocado oil
- 1 cup cherry tomatoes, halved
- 3 scallions, chopped
- ½ teaspoon turmeric powder
- Juice of 1 lime
- Salt and black pepper to the taste
- 1 tablespoon chives, chopped

Directions:

1. Heat up a pan with the oil over medium heat, add the scallions and the turmeric and cook for 2 minutes.
2. Add the tuna and the other ingredients, toss gently, cook for 12 minutes more, divide between plates and serve.

Nutrition:

calories 150, fat 3, fiber 6, carbs 3, protein 8

Ginger and Cumin Salmon

Prep time: 5 minutes | **Cooking time:** 14 minutes | **Servings:** 2

Ingredients:

- 1 pound salmon fillets, boneless and cubed
- 1 teaspoon sweet paprika
- 1 tablespoon olive oil
- ½ teaspoon cumin, ground
- 2 teaspoons ginger, grated
- Juice of 1 lime
- A pinch of salt and black pepper

Directions:

1. Heat up a pan with the oil over medium heat, add the ginger and the other ingredients except the salmon and cook for 4 minutes.
2. Add the salmon, cook for 10 minutes more, divide everything between plates and serve.

Nutrition:

calories 80, fat 6, fiber 1, carbs 2, protein 4

Coconut Cream Shrimps

Prep time: 5 minutes | **Cooking time:** 10 minutes | **Servings:** 2

Ingredients:

- 1 pound shrimp, peeled and deveined
- 1 tablespoon avocado oil
- 3 scallions, minced
- 2 garlic cloves, minced
- A pinch of salt and black pepper
- 1 teaspoon hot paprika
- 1 cup coconut cream

Directions:

1. Heat up a pan with the oil over medium heat, add the scallions and the garlic and cook for 2 minutes.
2. Add the shrimp and the other ingredients, toss, cook for 8 minutes more, divide into bowls and serve.

Nutrition:

calories 455, fat 6, fiber 5, carbs 4, protein 13

Vegetables with Calamari

Prep time: 5 minutes | **Cooking time:** 20 minutes | **Servings:** 2

Ingredients:

- 1 pound calamari rings
- 1 tablespoon olive oil
- 1 shallot, chopped
- 2 garlic cloves, minced
- 1 cup radishes, halved
- 1 cup baby spinach
- ½ cup chicken broth
- 1 tablespoon cilantro, chopped
- A pinch of salt and black pepper

Directions:

1. Heat up a pan with the oil over medium heat, add the shallot and the garlic and cook for 2 minutes.
2. Add the calamari rings and the other ingredients, toss, cook for 18 minutes more, divide between plates and serve.

Nutrition:

calories 300, fat 12, fiber 2, carbs 6, protein 20

Perfect Keto Tuna

Prep time: 10 minutes | **Cooking time:** 14 minutes | **Servings:** 2

Ingredients:

- 1 tablespoon olive oil
- 1 pound tuna fillets, boneless and cubed
- 1 tablespoon ginger, grated
- ½ teaspoon cumin, ground
- ½ teaspoon coriander, ground
- A pinch of salt and black pepper
- ½ tablespoon chives, chopped

Directions:

1. Heat up a pot with the oil over medium heat, add the add the ginger, cumin and coriander and cook for 4 minutes.
2. Add the tuna and the rest of the ingredients, toss, cook for 10 minutes more, divide into bowls and serve.

Nutrition:

calories 200, fat 3, fiber 2, carbs 4, protein 14

Shrimps and Bell Peppers Bowl

Prep time: 5 minutes | **Cooking time:** 12 minutes | **Servings:** 2

Ingredients:

- 1 pound shrimp, peeled and deveined
- 1 red bell pepper, cut into strips
- 1 green bell pepper, cut into strips
- 1 tablespoon olive oil
- 2 garlic cloves, minced
- 2 tablespoons lime juice
- 1 tablespoon parsley, chopped

Directions:

1. Heat up a pan with the oil over medium heat, add the garlic and peppers and cook for 4 minutes.
2. Add the shrimp and the other ingredients, toss, cook for 7 minutes more, divide into bowls and serve.

Nutrition:

calories 50, fat 1, fiber 0, carbs 0.5, protein 2

Aromatic Trout

Prep time: 10 minutes | **Cooking time:** 20 minutes | **Servings:** 2

Ingredients:

- 2 trout fillets, boneless
- 1 tablespoon ghee, melted
- 3 scallions, chopped
- 1 tablespoon rosemary, chopped
- ¼ cup chicken broth
- A pinch of salt and black pepper
- 1 tablespoon chives, chopped

Directions:

1. In a roasting pan, combine the trout with the ghee and the other ingredients, and bake at 390 degrees F for 20 minutes.
2. Divide the trout mix between plates and serve.

Nutrition:

calories 200, fat 5, fiber 2, carbs 2, protein 7

Fish with Mustard Sauce

Prep time: 10 minutes | **Cooking time:** 20 minutes | **Servings:** 2

Ingredients:

- 2 salmon fillets, boneless and cubed
- 2 tablespoons ghee, melted
- 1 tablespoon mustard
- 1 tablespoon lime juice
- A pinch of salt and black pepper
- ½ teaspoon cumin, ground
- ½ teaspoon coriander, ground
- 3 scallions, chopped

Directions:

1. Heat up a pan with the ghee over medium heat, add the mustard and the other ingredients except the salmon, stir and cook for 5 minutes.
2. Add the fish, cook for 15 minutes more, divide into bowls and serve.

Nutrition:

calories 240, fat 7, fiber 1, carbs 5, protein 23

Salmon with Halved Tomatoes

Prep time: 10 minutes | **Cooking time:** 20 minutes

Servings: 2

Ingredients:

- 2 salmon fillets, boneless
- 1 cup cherry tomatoes, halved
- 1 tablespoon olive oil
- 1 tablespoon parsley, chopped
- A pinch of salt and black pepper
- 2 scallions, chopped
- 1 tablespoon lemon juice

Directions:

1. Heat up a pan with the oil over medium heat, add the scallions and cook for 2 minutes.
2. Add the fish and cook it for 10 minutes.
3. Add the tomatoes and the remaining ingredients, toss, cook for 8 minutes more, divide between plates and serve.

Nutrition:

calories 200, fat 10, fiber 1, carbs 5, protein 20

Thyme Seafood Bowl

Prep time: 10 minutes | **Cooking time:** 12 minutes | **Servings:** 2

Ingredients:

- 1 pound shrimp, peeled and deveined
- 1 tablespoon olive oil
- 1 teaspoon thyme, ground
- 4 scallions, chopped
- 1 cup tomato passata (unsweetened)
- A pinch of salt and black pepper
- ½ teaspoon sweet paprika

Directions:

1. Heat up a pan with the oil over medium heat, add the scallions and the paprika and cook for 4 minutes.
2. Add the shrimp and the other ingredients, toss, cook for 8 minutes more, divide into bowls and serve.

Nutrition:

calories 420, fat 22, fiber 0, carbs 5, protein 25

Marjoram Seafood Bowl

Prep time: 5 minutes | **Cooking time:** 8 minutes | **Servings:** 2

Ingredients:

- 1 pound shrimp, peeled and deveined
- 1 tablespoon olive oil
- ½ teaspoon sweet paprika
- ½ teaspoon garam masala
- 1 tablespoon marjoram, chopped
- ¼ cup chicken broth
- A pinch of salt and black pepper
- 3 garlic cloves, minced

Directions:

1. Heat up a pan with the oil over medium heat, add the garlic and cook for 2 minutes.
2. Add the shrimp and the other ingredients, toss, cook for 6 minutes more, divide into bowls and serve.

Nutrition:

calories 136, fat 5, fiber 0, carbs 1, protein 20

Garlic Mussels

Prep time: 10 minutes | **Cooking time:** 15 minutes | **Servings:** 2

Ingredients:

- 1 pounds mussels
- 1 tablespoon ghee, melted
- 3 scallions, chopped
- 1 cup chicken broth
- 1 teaspoon red pepper flakes, crushed
- 3 garlic cloves, minced
- 1 handful parsley, chopped
- A pinch of salt and black pepper

Directions:

1. Heat up a pan with the ghee over medium heat, add the scallions and garlic and cook for 2 minutes.
2. Add the mussels and the other ingredients, toss, cook for 13 minutes more, divide into bowls and serve.

Nutrition:

calories 250, fat 3, fiber 3, carbs 2, protein 8

Tarragon and Cumin Swordfish Steaks

Prep time: 5 minutes | **Cooking time:** 8 minutes | **Servings:** 2

Ingredients:

- 2 swordfish steaks
- A pinch of salt and black pepper
- 1 tablespoon olive oil
- 1 tablespoon tarragon, chopped
- Juice of 1 lime
- ½ teaspoon cumin
- ¼ teaspoon garlic powder

Directions:

1. 1. Heat up a pan with the oil over medium high eat, add the swordfish steaks, salt, pepper and the other ingredients, toss, cook for 4 minutes on each side, divide between plates and serve with a side salad.

Nutrition:

calories 160, fat 3, fiber 2, carbs 4, protein 8

Baked Cod with Parsley

Prep time: 10 minutes | **Cooking time:** 20 minutes | **Servings:** 2

Ingredients:

- 2 cod fillets, boneless
- 2 tablespoons ghee, melted
- 1 tablespoon balsamic vinegar
- 2 teaspoons garam masala
- 2 tablespoons parsley, chopped
- A pinch of salt and black pepper

Directions:

1. In a roasting pan, combine the cod fillets with the ghee and the other ingredients, toss, introduce in the oven at 370 degrees F and bake for 20 minutes.
2. Divide between plates and serve with a side salad.

Nutrition:

calories 150, fat 3, fiber 2, carbs 0.7, protein 4

Sea Bass and Baby Kale Bowl

Prep time: 10 minutes | **Cooking time:** 20 minutes | **Servings:** 2

Ingredients:

- 2 sea bass fillets, boneless
- 2 scallions, chopped
- 1 cup baby kale
- 1 cup tomato passata (unsweetened)
- 1 tablespoon avocado oil
- A pinch of salt and black pepper
- Juice of 1 lime
- 1 tablespoon chives, chopped

Directions:

1. Heat up a pan with the oil over medium heat, add the scallions and the kale and cook for 5 minutes.
2. Add the fish and the rest of the ingredients, toss gently, cook over medium heat for 15 minutes more, divide between plates and serve.

Nutrition:

calories 240, fat 7.5, fiber 3, carbs 5.3, protein 10

Tender Fish and Cabbage Salad

Prep time: 10 minutes | **Servings:** 2

Ingredients:

- 1 pound smoked salmon, skinless, boneless and cut into strips
- 1 red cabbage head, shredded
- 2 spring onions, chopped
- 2 tablespoons olive oil
- Juice of 1 lime
- 3 scallions, chopped
- A pinch of salt and black pepper
- ½ cup kalamata olives, pitted and halved
- ¼ cup pepitas, toasted

Directions:

1. 1. In a bowl, combine the salmon with the cabbage and the other ingredients, toss and serve.

Nutrition:

calories 160, fat 6, fiber 1, carbs 1, protein 12

Spiced Tuna Fillets

Prep time: 5 minutes | **Cooking time:** 10 minutes | **Servings:** 2

Ingredients:

- 1 pound tuna fillets, boneless
- 4 green onions, chopped
- 1 tablespoon avocado oil
- A pinch of salt and black pepper
- 1 tablespoon lemon juice
- ½ teaspoon cumin, ground
- ½ teaspoon chili powder

Directions:

1. 1. Heat up a pan with the oil over medium heat, add the tuna fillets, green onions and the other ingredients, cook them for 5 minutes on each side, divide between plates and serve.

Nutrition:

calories 300, fat 12, fiber 6, carbs 6, protein 15

Keto Crackers

Prep time: 10 minutes | **Cooking time:** 20 minutes | **Servings:** 2

Ingredients:

- 2 cups flax seed, soaked overnight and drained
- 4 bunches kale, chopped
- 1 tablespoon lime juice
- 4 garlic cloves, minced
- 1/3 cup olive oil

Directions:

1. In your food processor combine the flaxseed with the kale and the other ingredients and pulse well.
2. Spread this into a tray, cut into medium crackers, introduce in the oven and cook at 400 degrees F for 20 minutes.
3. Arrange them on a platter and serve.

Nutrition:

calories 100, fat 1, fiber 2, carbs 1, protein 4

Chili Dip

Prep time: 10 minutes | **Cooking time:** 20 minutes | **Servings:** 2

Ingredients:

- 1 cup spring onions, chopped
- 1 tablespoon chives, chopped
- ¾ cup cream cheese, soft
- ½ cup coconut cream
- ½ teaspoon chili powder
- ½ teaspoon cumin, ground
- ½ teaspoon garlic powder
- A pinch of salt and black pepper

Directions:

1. 1. In a pan, combine the cream with the spring onions, chives and the other ingredients, whisk, cook over medium heat for 20 minutes, divide into bowls and serve.

Nutrition:

calories 60, fat 4, fiber 1, carbs 1, protein 1

Mint and Garlic Shrimp

Prep time: 5 minutes | **Cooking time:** 8 minutes | **Servings:** 2

Ingredients:

- 1 pound shrimp, peeled and deveined
- 1 tablespoon ghee, melted
- 1 tablespoon mint, chopped
- 1 tablespoon garlic, minced
- ½ teaspoon red pepper flakes
- ½ teaspoon hot paprika
- 1 tablespoon parsley, chopped

Directions:

1. Heat up a pan with the oil over medium high heat, add the garlic, pepper flakes and paprika and cook for 2 minutes.
2. Add the shrimp and the other ingredients, toss, cook for 6 minutes more, divide the mix into bowls and serve,

Nutrition:

calories 150, fat 3, fiber 3, carbs 1, protein 7

Ketogenic Poultry Recipes

Turmeric Chicken

Prep time: 10 minutes | **Cooking time:** 20 minutes | **Servings:** 2

Ingredients:

- 2 chicken breasts, skinless boneless and sliced
- 3 scallions, chopped
- A pinch of salt and black pepper
- 1 tablespoon olive oil
- 1 tablespoon ghee, melted
- ½ teaspoon turmeric powder
- ½ teaspoon coriander, ground
- ½ cup chicken broth
- 2 tablespoons cilantro, chopped

Directions:

1. Heat up a pan with the oil and the ghee over medium heat, add the scallions and cook for 2 minutes.
2. Add the meat and cook it for 3 minutes more.
3. Add the rest of the ingredients, toss, cook for 15 minutes more, divide between plates and serve.

Nutrition:

calories 128, fat 13.6, fiber 0.8, carbs 2.3, protein 0.7

Coriander Turkey Bowl

Prep time: 10 minutes | **Cooking time:** 30 minutes | **Servings:** 2

Ingredients:

- 1 pound turkey breast, skinless, boneless and cut into strips
- 2 tablespoons ghee, melted
- 3 scallions, chopped
- 3 garlic cloves, minced
- ½ cup cherry tomatoes, halved
- 1 cup zucchinis, cubed
- 1 red bell pepper, cubed
- A pinch of salt and black pepper
- 1 tablespoon coriander, ground
- 1 tablespoon cilantro, chopped

Directions:

1. Heat up a pan with the ghee over medium heat, add the scallions and garlic and cook for 5 minutes.
2. Add the meat and cook for 5 minutes more.
3. Add the other ingredients, toss, cook for 20 minutes more, divide everything into bowls and serve.

Nutrition:

calories 240, fat 4, fiber 3, carbs 2, protein 12

Tender Chicken Cubes with Kalamata Olives

Prep time: 10 minutes | **Cooking time:** 30 minutes | **Servings:** 2

Ingredients:

- 1 pound chicken breast, skinless, boneless and cubed
- ½ cup kalamata olives, pitted and halved
- 1 tablespoon olive oil
- 2 shallots, chopped
- 1 cup cheddar cheese, shredded
- A pinch of salt and black pepper
- 1 tablespoon cilantro, chopped
- ¼ teaspoon cumin, ground
- ½ teaspoon coriander, ground

Directions:

1. Heat up a pan with the oil over medium heat, add the shallots, cumin and coriander and cook for 5 minutes.
2. Add the meat and cook for 5 minutes more.
3. Add the rest of the ingredients, toss, cook for 20 minutes more, divide everything between plates and serve.

Nutrition:

calories 223, fat 8, fiber 1, carbs 3, protein 26

Chicken with Curry Paste and Coconut Cream

Prep time: 10 minutes | **Cooking time:** 25 minutes | **Servings:** 2

Ingredients:

- 1 pound chicken breast, skinless, boneless and cubed
- 1 tablespoon ghee, melted
- 1 cup chicken broth
- ¼ cup coconut cream
- 2 scallions, chopped
- 1 cup celery stalk, chopped
- 1 tablespoon yellow curry paste
- A pinch of salt and black pepper

Directions:

1. Heat up a pan with the ghee over medium heat, add the scallions and curry paste and cook for 5 minutes.
2. Add the meat and brown for 5 minutes more.
3. Add the rest of the ingredients, toss, cook for 15 minutes, divide into bowls and serve.

Nutrition:

calories 120, fat 2, fiber 2, carbs 6, protein 10

Poultry Stir Fry

Prep time: 10 minutes | **Cooking time:** 20 minutes | **Servings:** 2

Ingredients:

- 1 pound turkey breast, skinless, boneless and cubed
- 1 cup cherry tomatoes, halved
- 1 zucchini, cubed
- 1 green bell pepper, cubed
- 1 tablespoon olive oil
- ½ teaspoon sweet paprika
- ½ teaspoon coriander, ground
- 1 cup baby spinach
- 1 teaspoon red pepper flakes, crushed
- 1 teaspoon onion powder
- 1 tablespoon ginger, grated
- 1 tablespoon chives, chopped

Directions:

1. Heat up a pan with the oil over medium heat, add the meat and brown for 5 minutes.
2. Add the cherry tomatoes and the other ingredients except the spinach, toss and cook for 15 minutes.
3. Add the spinach, toss, cook for 5 minutes more.
4. Divide the mix into bowls and serve.

Nutrition:

calories 210, fat 10, fiber 3, carbs 5, protein 20

Rosemary Chicken with Artichokes

Prep time: 10 minutes | **Cooking time:** 25 minutes | **Servings:** 2

Ingredients:

- 1 pound chicken breast, skinless, boneless and cubed
- 2 artichoke hearts, trimmed and quartered
- 1 cup kalamata olives, pitted and halved
- 2 tablespoons ghee, melted
- ½ teaspoon sweet paprika
- ½ teaspoon rosemary, dried
- A pinch of salt and black pepper
- ¼ cup chicken broth
- 1 tablespoon cilantro, chopped

Directions:

1. Heat up a pan with the ghee over medium heat, add the meat and brown for 5 minutes.
2. Add the artichokes and the other ingredients, toss, cook for 20 minutes more, divide between plates and serve.

Nutrition:

calories 450, fat 23, fiber 1, carbs 3, protein 39

Tender Chicken and Greens

Prep time: 10 minutes | **Cooking time:** 30 minutes | **Servings:** 2

Ingredients:
- 1 pound chicken breast, skinless, boneless and cubed
- 2 cups mustard greens, torn
- 1 tablespoon olive oil
- 3 scallions, chopped
- 1 red bell pepper, chopped
- 2 garlic cloves, minced
- A pinch of salt and black pepper
- ½ cup chicken broth
- 1 tablespoon cilantro, chopped

Directions:
1. Heat up a pan with the oil over medium heat, add the scallions, garlic and the bell pepper and cook for 5 minutes.
2. Add the meat and brown for 5 minutes more.
3. Add the rest of the ingredients, toss, cook for 20 minutes more, divide everything between plates and serve.

Nutrition:
calories 340, fat 33, fiber 3, carbs 4, protein 20

Herbs and Chicken Mix

Prep time: 10 minutes | **Cooking time:** 20 minutes | **Servings:** 2

Ingredients:
- 1 pound chicken breast, skinless, boneless and cubed
- 1 tablespoon ghee, melted
- 2 avocados, peeled, pitted and cubed
- 2 spring onions, chopped
- ½ cup chicken broth
- A pinch of salt and black pepper
- 1 teaspoon oregano, dried
- 1 tablespoon cilantro, chopped

Directions:
1. Heat up a pan with the ghee over medium heat, add the spring onions and cook for 2 minutes.
2. Add the chicken and brown for 3 minutes more.
3. Add the rest of the ingredients, toss, cook for 15 minutes, divide the mix between plates and serve.

Nutrition:
calories 300, fat 6, fiber 3, carbs 5, protein 28

Shredded Cabbage and Chicken Mix

Prep time: 10 minutes | **Cooking time:** 25 minutes | **Servings:** 2

Ingredients:
- 1 pound chicken breast, skinless, boneless and cubed
- 1 Savoy cabbage, shredded
- 2 tablespoons avocado oil
- 1 cup tomato passata (unsweetened)
- 2 shallots, chopped
- 1 teaspoon chili powder
- ½ teaspoon coriander, ground
- A pinch of salt and black pepper
- 1 tablespoon cilantro, chopped

Directions:
1. Heat up a pan with the oil over medium high heat, add the shallots, chili powder and coriander and cook for 5 minutes.
2. Add the chicken and cook for 5 minutes more.
3. Add the rest of the ingredients, toss, cook for 15 minutes, divide into bowls and serve.

Nutrition:
calories 290, fat 12, fiber 2, carbs 4, protein 24

Garam Masala Chicken

Prep time: 10 minutes | **Cooking time:** 20 minutes | **Servings:** 2

Ingredients:
- 1 tablespoon olive oil
- 1 pound chicken breast, skinless, boneless and cubed
- 2 scallions, minced
- 2 garlic cloves, minced
- ½ teaspoon garam masala
- ¼ cup coconut milk
- 2 tablespoons cilantro, chopped
- A pinch of salt and black pepper

Directions:
1. Heat up a pan with the oil over medium high heat, add the scallions and garlic and cook for 2 minutes.
2. Add the meat and brown for 3 minutes more.
3. Add the rest of the ingredients, toss, cook for 15 minutes, divide into bowls and serve.

Nutrition:
calories 112, fat 7.9, fiber 0.6, carbs 3, protein 7.9

Oregano Turkey

Prep time: 10 minutes | **Cooking time:** 25 minutes | **Servings:** 2

Ingredients:
- 1 pound turkey breast, skinless, boneless and cubed
- 2 tablespoons ghee, melted
- 2 teaspoons cumin, ground
- ½ teaspoon oregano, dried
- 2 scallions, chopped
- A pinch of salt and black pepper
- 1 tablespoon cilantro, chopped

Directions:
1. Heat up the pan with the ghee over medium heat, add the scallions and cook for 2 minutes.
2. Add the meat and brown for 3 minutes more.
3. Add the rest of the ingredients, toss, cook for 20 minutes more, divide between plates and serve.

Nutrition:
calories 240, fat 10, fiber 2, carbs 5, protein 20

Red Chili Pepper Turkey

Prep time: 10 minutes | **Cooking time:** 30 minutes | **Servings:** 2

Ingredients:
- 1 pound turkey breast, skinless, boneless and cubed
- 1 teaspoon chili powder
- ½ teaspoon hot paprika
- 1 red chili pepper, minced
- 2 spring onions, chopped
- 1 tablespoon olive oil
- 1 cup chicken broth
- 1 tablespoon chives, chopped

Directions:
1. Heat up a pan with the oil over medium heat, add the spring onions and chili pepper and cook for 5 minutes.
2. Add the meat and brown for 5 minutes more.
3. Add the rest of the ingredients, toss, cook for 20 minutes, divide between plates and serve.

Nutrition:
calories 360, fat 32, fiber 2, carbs 7, protein 20

Zucchini and Ground Chicken Bowl

Prep time: 10 minutes

Cooking time: 20 minutes | **Servings:** 2

Ingredients:

- 1 pound chicken breast, skinless, boneless and ground
- 1 tablespoon olive oil
- 1 zucchini, cubed
- 1 avocado, peeled, pitted and cubed
- 2 scallions, chopped
- 1 cup cherry tomatoes, cubed
- 2 tablespoon lime juice
- A pinch of salt and black pepper
- 1 tablespoon chives, chopped

Directions:

1. Heat up a pan with the oil over medium heat, add the scallions and cook for 2 minutes.
2. Add the meat and brown for 3 minutes more.
3. Add the rest of the ingredients, toss, cook for 15 minutes more, divide everything into bowls and serve.

Nutrition:

calories 120, fat 2, fiber 1, carbs 3, protein 7

Leek and Turkey

Prep time: 10 minutes | Cooking time: 30 minutes | **Servings:** 2

Ingredients:

- 1 pound turkey breast, skinless, boneless and cubed
- 2 leeks, sliced
- ½ cup shallots, chopped
- 2 tablespoons ghee, melted
- 2 garlic cloves, minced
- 1 cup chicken broth
- ½ cup tomato passata (unsweetened)
- 1 tablespoon parsley, chopped
- A pinch of salt and black pepper

Directions:

1. Heat up a pan with the ghee over medium-high heat, add the shallots and the garlic and cook for 5 minutes.
2. Add the meat and brown for 5 minutes more.
3. Add the rest of the ingredients, toss, cook for 20 minutes more, divide between plates and serve.

Nutrition:

calories 240, fat 4, fiber 3, carbs 6, protein 20

Coriander Chicken with Fennel

Prep time: 10 minutes | Cooking time: 25 minutes | **Servings:** 2

Ingredients:

- 2 tablespoons olive oil
- 1 pound chicken breast, skinless, boneless and cubed
- 1 fennel bulb, sliced
- 2 garlic cloves, minced
- 1 cup tomato passata
- (unsweetened)
- ½ teaspoon coriander, ground
- A pinch of salt and black pepper
- 1 tablespoon cilantro, chopped

Directions:

1. Heat up a pan with the oil over medium heat, garlic and the meat and cook for 5 minutes.
2. Add the fennel and the other ingredients, toss, cook for 20 minutes more, divide into bowls and serve.

Nutrition:

calories 400, fat 23, fiber 5, carbs 5, protein 30

Cauliflower Florets with Ginger Chicken

Prep time: 10 minutes | Cooking time: 25 minutes | **Servings:** 2

Ingredients:

- 1 pound chicken thighs, boneless, skinless and cubed
- 1 cup cauliflower florets
- 1 tablespoon olive oil
- A pinch of salt and black pepper
- 1 tablespoon ginger, grated
- 1 tablespoon lime juice
- A pinch of red pepper flakes
- Salt and black pepper to the taste
- 2 garlic cloves, minced
- 2 scallions, chopped
- ½ teaspoon rosemary, dried
- 1 teaspoon sweet paprika

Directions:

1. Heat up a pan with the oil over medium heat, add the garlic and the scallions and cook for 5 minutes.
2. Add the meat and brown for 5 minutes.
3. Add the rest of the ingredients, toss, cook for 15 minutes more, divide between plates and serve.

Nutrition:

calories 375, fat 12, fiber 1, carbs 3, protein 42

Cumin and Coconut Cream Chicken Breast

Prep time: 10 minutes | Cooking time: 25 minutes | **Servings:** 2

Ingredients:

- 1 pound chicken breast, skinless, boneless and cubed
- 2 tablespoons ghee, melted
- 1 tablespoon thyme, chopped
- 3 garlic cloves, minced
- ½ cup coconut cream
- A pinch of salt and black pepper
- ½ teaspoon cumin, ground

Directions:

1. Heat up a pan with the ghee over medium heat, add the garlic and the meat and brown for 5 minutes.
2. Add the rest of the ingredients, toss, cook for 20 minutes more, divide everything between plates and serve.

Nutrition:

calories 224, fat 11, fiber 4, carbs 6, protein 23

Sesame and Ginger Chicken

Prep time: 10 minutes | Cooking time: 25 minutes | **Servings:** 2

Ingredients:

- 1 pound chicken breast, skinless, boneless and cubed
- A pinch of salt and black pepper
- 2 tablespoons ghee, melted
- ½ teaspoon turmeric powder
- 1 tablespoon sesame seeds
- 1 tablespoon ginger, grated
- 2 tablespoons scallions, chopped
- 1 tablespoon cilantro, chopped

Directions:

1. Heat up a pan with the ghee over medium heat, add the scallions and the ginger and cook for 2 minutes.
2. Add the chicken and brown for 3 minutes more.
3. Add the rest of the ingredients, toss, cook for 20 minutes, divide into bowls and serve.

Nutrition:

calories 423, fat 20, fiber 5, carbs 6, protein 45

Vegetables and Chicken Strips

Prep time: 10 minutes | **Cooking time:** 20 minutes | **Servings:** 2

Ingredients:

- 1 pound chicken breast, skinless, boneless and cut into strips
- 1 cup baby kale
- 1 tablespoon olive oil
- ½ teaspoon coriander, ground
- ½ teaspoon rosemary, dried
- A pinch of salt and black pepper
- 1 cup tomato passata (unsweetened)
- 1 tablespoon cilantro, chopped

Directions:

1. Heat up a pan with the oil over medium heat, add the chicken and cook for 5 minutes.
2. Add the kale and the other ingredients, toss, cook for 15 minutes more, divide between plates and serve.

Nutrition:

calories 260, fat 5, fiber 1, carbs 2, protein 20

Green Beans and Turkey

Prep time: 10 minutes | **Cooking time:** 30 minutes | **Servings:** 2

Ingredients:

- 1 pound chicken breasts, skinless, boneless and cubed
- 1 cup green beans, trimmed and halved
- 1 cup cherry tomatoes, halved
- 2 tablespoons olive oil
- 1 tablespoon chives, chopped
- ½ teaspoon sweet paprika
- 1 teaspoon garlic powder
- A pinch of salt and black pepper

Directions:

1. Heat up a pan with the oil over medium heat, add the meat and brown for 5 minutes.
2. Add the green beans and the other ingredients, toss, cook for 25 minutes more, divide between plates and serve.

Nutrition:

calories 340, fat 8, fiber 2, carbs 6, protein 20

Cheddar Chicken Thighs

Prep time: 10 minutes | **Cooking time:** 25 minutes | **Servings:** 2

Ingredients:

- 1 pound chicken tights, skinless, boneless
- 1 cup cheddar cheese, shredded
- 1 tablespoon ghee, melted
- A pinch of salt and black pepper
- 1 cup chicken broth
- 1 teaspoon basil, dried
- 1 teaspoon chili powder
- 2 jalapenos, chopped

Directions:

1. Heat up a pan with the ghee over medium heat, add the chicken and brown for 5 minutes.
2. Add the rest of the ingredients except the cheese and toss.
3. Sprinkle the cheese on top and bake at 400 degrees F for 20 minutes more.
4. Divide everything between plates and serve.

Nutrition:

calories 400, fat 22, fiber 3, carbs 6, protein 38

Mustard and Garlic Chicken

Prep time: 10 minutes | **Cooking time:** 25 minutes | **Servings:** 2

Ingredients:

- 1 pound chicken breast, skinless, boneless and cubed
- 3 scallions, chopped
- 2 tablespoons ghee, melted
- 1 tablespoon ginger, grated
- ½ cup chicken broth
- 3 garlic cloves, minced
- A pinch of salt and black pepper
- 2 tablespoons Dijon mustard
- 1 tablespoon chives, chopped

Directions:

1. Heat up a pan with the ghee over medium heat, add the scallions, ginger and garlic and cook for 5 minutes.
2. Add the chicken and brown for 5 minutes more.
3. Add the rest of the ingredients, toss, cook for 15 minutes more, divide between plates and serve.

Nutrition:

calories 600, fat 54, fiber 14, carbs 10, protein 45

Basil and Garlic Chicken

Prep time: 10 minutes | **Cooking time:** 30 minutes | **Servings:** 2

Ingredients:

- 1 pound chicken breast, skinless, boneless and sliced
- 1 teaspoon Italian seasoning
- ¼ cup chicken broth
- 2 garlic cloves, minced
- 1 tablespoon olive oil
- A pinch of salt and black pepper
- 1 teaspoon garlic powder
- ½ teaspoon basil, dried
- ½ tablespoon chives, chopped

Directions:

1. Heat up a pan with the oil over medium heat, add the meat and garlic and brown for 5 minutes.
2. Add the rest of the ingredients, toss, introduce in the oven and cook at 390 degrees F for 25 minutes more.
3. Divide everything between plates and serve.

Nutrition:

calories 235, fat 4, fiber 1, carbs 2, protein 35

Chicken with Endives

Prep time: 10 minutes | **Cooking time:** 25 minutes | **Servings:** 2

Ingredients:

- 1 pound chicken wings
- A pinch of salt and black pepper
- 1 tablespoon ghee, melted
- 2 endives, shredded
- 1 tablespoon balsamic vinegar
- ¼ cup scallions, chopped
- ½ teaspoon coriander, ground
- ½ teaspoon sweet paprika
- 1 tablespoon cilantro, chopped

Directions:

1. Heat up a pan with the ghee over medium heat, add the scallions and the endives and cook for 5 minutes.
2. Add the meat and brown for 5 minutes more.
3. Add the rest of the ingredients, toss, cook for 15 minutes more, divide between plates and serve.

Nutrition:

calories 415, fat 23, fiber 3, carbs 2, protein 27

Bella Mushrooms and Turkey

Prep time: 10 minutes | **Cooking time:** 30 minutes | **Servings:** 2

Ingredients:

- 1 pound turkey breast, skinless, boneless and cubed
- 2 tablespoons ghee, melted
- 1 cup baby Bella mushrooms, halved
- 1 teaspoon sweet paprika
- ½ teaspoon coriander, ground
- ½ teaspoon rosemary, dried
- A pinch of salt and black pepper
- ½ cup coconut cream
- 1 tablespoon cilantro, chopped

Directions:

1. Heat up a pan with the ghee over medium heat, add the meat and brown for 5 minutes.
2. Add the mushrooms and cook for 5 minutes more.
3. Add the rest of the ingredients, toss, cook for 20 minutes more, divide between plates and serve.

Nutrition:

calories 200, fat 4, fiber 1, carbs 2, protein 7

Chicken in Tender Sauce

Prep time: 10 minutes | **Cooking time:** 25 minutes | **Servings:** 2

Ingredients:

- 1 pound chicken breasts, skinless, boneless and cubed
- ½ cup shallots, minced
- 2 tablespoons ghee, melted
- ½ cup chicken broth
- ¼ cup parsley, chopped
- 1 tablespoons lime juice
- A pinch of salt and black pepper
- ½ teaspoon coriander, ground

Directions:

1. Heat up a pan with the ghee over medium heat, add the shallots and lime juice, stir and cook for 10 minutes.
2. Add the meat and brown for 5 minutes.
3. Add the rest of the ingredients, toss, cook for 10 minutes more, divide between plates and serve.

Nutrition:

calories 230, fat 12, fiber 5.0, carbs 6.3, protein 20

Parmesan Chicken with Radish

Prep time: 10 minutes | **Cooking time:** 25 minutes | **Servings:** 2

Ingredients:

- 2 tablespoons ghee, melted
- 1 pound chicken thighs, boneless and skinless
- 1 cup radishes, halved
- ¼ cup chicken broth1
- ½ teaspoon sweet paprika
- 2 tablespoons parmesan, grated
- A pinch of salt and black pepper
- 2 garlic cloves, minced
- 1 tablespoon chives, chopped

Directions:

1. Heat up a pan the ghee over medium heat, add the garlic and the meat and brown for 5 minutes.
2. Add the rest of the ingredients except the parmesan and toss.
3. Sprinkle the cheese on top and cook for 20 minutes more.
4. Divide everything between plates and serve.

Nutrition:

calories 340, fat 31, fiber 3, carbs 5, protein 64

Chicken Roast

Prep time: 10 minutes | **Cooking time:** 30 minutes | **Servings:** 2

Ingredients:

- 1 pound chicken breasts, skinless, boneless and halved
- 1 tablespoon olive oil
- 1 teaspoon smoked paprika
- ½ teaspoon onion powder
- ½ teaspoon garlic powder
- A pinch of salt and black pepper
- 1 tablespoon rosemary, chopped
- 1 tablespoon basil, chopped
- 1 teaspoon Italian seasoning
- ¼ cup chicken broth

Directions:

1. Grease a baking dish with the oil, and add the chicken breasts inside.
2. Add the rest of the ingredients, toss, cook at 390 degrees F for 30 minutes, divide between plates and serve.

Nutrition:

calories 450, fat 30, fiber 1, carbs 1, protein 34

Garam Masala Duck

Prep time: 10 minutes | **Cooking time:** 25 minutes | **Servings:** 2

Ingredients:

- 2 tablespoons ghee, melted
- 1 pound duck breast, skinless, boneless and cut into strips
- 4 green onions, chopped
- ½ teaspoon coriander, ground
- ½ teaspoon garam masala
- ½ teaspoon turmeric powder
- ¼ cup chicken broth
- A pinch of salt and black pepper

Directions:

1. Heat up a pan with the ghee over medium high heat, add the green onions and cook for 5 minutes.
2. Add the meat and the other ingredients, toss, cook for 20 minutes, divide everything into bowls and serve.

Nutrition:

calories 200, fat 7, fiber 2, carbs 1, protein 8

Lemon Turkey Bowl

Prep time: 10 minutes | **Cooking time:** 30 minutes | **Servings:** 2

Ingredients:

- 2 avocados, peeled, pitted and cubed
- 1 pound turkey breast, skinless, boneless and cubed
- 1 cup baby spinach
- 3 scallions, chopped
- 1 tablespoon olive oil
- Juice of ½ lemon
- A pinch of salt and black pepper
- ½ teaspoon sweet paprika
- ½ teaspoon cumin, ground
- 1 teaspoon thyme, dried

Directions:

1. Heat up a pan with the oil over medium heat, add the scallions and cook for 2 minutes.
2. Add the meat and brown for 3 minutes more.
3. Add the rest of the ingredients, toss, cook for 25 minutes more, divide everything between plates and serve.

Nutrition:

calories 230, fat 40, fiber 11, carbs 5, protein 24

Mushrooms, Parsley, and Chicken Bowl

Prep time: 10 minutes | Cooking time: 25 minutes | Servings: 2

Ingredients:

- 1 pound chicken breast, skinless, boneless and cubed
- 1 cup mushrooms, halved
- 1 tablespoon ghee, melted
- A pinch of salt and black pepper
- 2 scallions, chopped
- 2 garlic cloves, minced
- 1 cup coconut cream
- A handful parsley, chopped

Directions:

1. Heat up a pan with the ghee over medium heat, add the scallions, garlic and the meat and brown for 5 minutes.
2. Add the rest of the ingredients, toss, cook for 20 minutes more, divide into bowls and serve.

Nutrition:

calories 340, fat 10, fiber 7, carbs 4, protein 24

Broccoli and Poultry Bowl

Prep time: 10 minutes | Cooking time: 25 minutes | Servings: 2

Ingredients:

- 3 scallions, chopped
- 1 pound turkey breast, skinless, boneless and cubed
- 2 tablespoons ghee, melted
- 1 cup broccoli florets
- ½ teaspoon sweet paprika
- 2 tablespoons balsamic vinegar
- ¼ cup chicken broth
- 1 tablespoon cilantro, chopped

Directions:

1. Heat up a pan with the ghee over medium heat, add the scallions and the paprika and cook for 5 minutes.
2. Add the turkey and brown for 5 minutes more.
3. Add the rest of the ingredients, toss, cook for 15 minutes, divide between plates and serve.

Nutrition:

calories 245, fat 13.40, fiber 4, carbs 5.6, protein 18

Spicy Chicken Breast Cubes

Prep time: 10 minutes | Cooking time: 20 minutes | Servings: 2

Ingredients:

- 1 pound chicken breast, skinless, boneless and cubed
- 2 tablespoons ghee, melted
- 3 scallions, chopped
- 2 cherry tomatoes, cubed
- 1 cup chicken broth
- A pinch of salt and black pepper
- ½ teaspoon allspice, ground
- 1 tablespoon chives, chopped

Directions:

1. Heat up a pan with the ghee over medium heat, add the meat and brown for 5 minutes.
2. Add the rest of the ingredients, toss, cook for 15 minutes more, divide between plates and serve.

Nutrition:

calories 407, fat 19, fiber 2.2, carbs 7.3, protein 50

Chives Chicken

Prep time: 10 minutes | Cooking time: 25 minutes | Servings: 2

Ingredients:

- 1 pound chicken breast, skinless, boneless and cubed
- 1 tablespoon ghee, melted
- 3 scallions, chopped
- 1 cup coconut cream
- 1 teaspoon turmeric powder
- 1 tablespoon chives, chopped
- A pinch of salt and black pepper

Directions:

1. Heat up a pan with the ghee over medium heat, add the scallions and cook for 5 minutes.
2. Add the meat and cook for 5 minutes more.
3. Add the rest of the ingredients, toss, cook for 15 minutes more, divide between plates and serve.

Nutrition:

calories 455, fat 20, fiber 0, carbs 2, protein 57

Mozzarella Chicken

Prep time: 10 minutes | Cooking time: 25 minutes | Servings: 2

Ingredients:

- 1 pound chicken breasts, skinless, boneless and cubed
- 1 tablespoon ghee, melted
- ½ cup cream cheese, soft
- 3 scallions, chopped
- Salt and black pepper to the taste
- 1 cup mozzarella, shredded
- ¼ teaspoon garlic powder
- 1 tablespoon chives, chopped

Directions:

1. Heat up a pan with the ghee over medium heat, add the scallions and garlic powder and cook for 2 minutes.
2. Add the chicken and brown for 3 minutes more.
3. Add the rest of the ingredients, toss, cook for 20 minutes more, divide into bowls and serve.

Nutrition:

calories 400, fat 22, fiber 1, carbs 1, protein 47

Ghee and Parmesan Chicken

Prep time: 10 minutes | Cooking time: 25 minutes | Servings: 2

Ingredients:

- 1 pound chicken breasts, skinless, boneless and cubed
- 2 tablespoons ghee, melted
- 1 tablespoon oregano, chopped
- 1 teaspoon turmeric powder
- 1 cup chicken broth
- 1 cup parmesan, grated
- A pinch of salt and black pepper

Directions:

1. Heat up a pan with the ghee over medium heat, add the oregano and turmeric and cook for 2 minutes.
2. Add the meat and brown for 3 minutes more.
3. Add the rest of the ingredients, toss, cook for 20 minutes more, divide between plates and serve.

Nutrition:

calories 250, fat 5, fiber 4, carbs 6, protein 25

Cheese Chicken

Prep time: 10 minutes | **Cooking time:** 25 minutes | **Servings:** 2

Ingredients:

- 1 pound chicken breast, skinless, boneless and sliced
- 1 tablespoon ghee, melted
- ½ teaspoon cumin, ground
- ½ teaspoon garam masala
- 1 tablespoon avocado oil
- A pinch of salt and black pepper
- 2 tablespoons parmesan, grated

Directions:

1. In a baking dish, combine the chicken with the ghee and the other ingredients except the parmesan and toss.
2. Sprinkle the parmesan on top and cook at 390 degrees F for 25 minutes.
3. Divide between plates and serve.

Nutrition:

calories 326, fat 13.1, fiber 0.4, carbs 0.7, protein 48.3

Scallions Chicken Cubes

Prep time: 10 minutes | **Cooking time:** 20 minutes | **Servings:** 2

Ingredients:

- 1 pound chicken breast, skinless, boneless and cubed
- 2 tablespoons ghee, melted
- 1 tablespoon sweet paprika
- 2 scallions, chopped
- ¼ cup chicken broth
- A pinch of salt and black pepper

Directions:

1. Heat up a pan with the ghee over medium heat, add the scallions and cook for 2 minutes.
2. Add the meat and brown for 3 minutes more.
3. Add the rest of the ingredients, toss and cook for 15 minutes.
4. Divide everything between plates and serve.

Nutrition:

calories 200, fat 6, fiber 3, carbs 6, protein 14

Radish Halves with Chicken Cubes

Prep time: 10 minutes | **Cooking time:** 25 minutes | **Servings:** 2

Ingredients:

- 1 pound chicken breast, skinless, boneless and cubed
- 1 tablespoon olive oil
- 1 cup radishes, halved
- 1 teaspoon turmeric powder
- ½ teaspoon chili powder
- A pinch of salt and black pepper
- 2 tablespoons parsley, chopped
- 2 garlic cloves, minced

Directions:

1. Heat up a pan with the oil over medium heat, add the meat and brown for 5 minutes.
2. Add the radishes and the other ingredients, toss, cook for 20 minutes more, divide into bowls and serve.

Nutrition:

calories 273, fat 14, fiber 1, carbs 4, protein 28

Garlic Turkey Breast with Brussels Sprouts

Prep time: 10 minutes | **Cooking time:** 25 minutes | **Servings:** 2

Ingredients:

- 2 tablespoons ghee, melted
- 1 pound turkey breast, skinless, boneless and cubed
- 1 cup Brussels sprouts, trimmed and halved
- 2 scallions, chopped
- 2 garlic cloves, minced
- A pinch of salt and black pepper
- ¼ teaspoon garlic powder
- 1 tablespoon chives, chopped

Directions:

1. Heat up a pan with the ghee over medium heat, add the scallions and garlic and cook for 2 minutes.
2. Add the meat and cook for 3 minutes more.
3. Add the rest of the ingredients, toss, cook for 20 minutes, divide between plates and serve.

Nutrition:

calories 320, fat 23, fiber 8, carbs 6, protein 16

Aromatic Spiced Turkey

Prep time: 10 minutes | **Cooking time:** 30 minutes | **Servings:** 2

Ingredients:

- 1 pound turkey breast, skinless, boneless and cubed
- 1 tablespoon olive oil
- 3 garlic cloves, minced
- A pinch of salt and black pepper
- 1 tablespoon balsamic vinegar
- 1 tablespoon basil, chopped
- ½ teaspoon chili powder
- 1 cup chicken broth

Directions:

1. Heat up a pan with the oil over medium high heat, add the garlic and the meat and brown for 5 minutes.
2. Add the rest of the ingredients, toss, cook for 25 minutes more, divide everything between plates and serve.

Nutrition:

calories 240, fat 12, fiber 1, carbs 4, protein 27

Nutmeg Chicken Cubes

Prep time: 10 minutes | **Cooking time:** 30 minutes | **Servings:** 2

Ingredients:

- 2 tablespoons ghee, melted
- 1 pound chicken breast, skinless, boneless and cubed
- 1 teaspoon nutmeg, ground
- A pinch of salt and black pepper
- 1 teaspoon garlic, minced
- 1 teaspoon Cajun seasoning
- ¼ cup scallions, chopped
- ½ cup chicken broth
- 1 tablespoon cilantro, chopped
- A pinch of salt and black pepper

Directions:

1. Heat up a pan with the ghee over medium heat, add the garlic and the scallions and cook for 5 minutes.
2. Add the meat and brown for 5 minutes more.
3. Add the rest of the ingredients, toss, cook for 20 minutes more, divide between plates and serve.

Nutrition:

calories 345, fat 34, fiber 4, carbs 4, protein 39

Asparagus and Tender Chicken Thighs

Prep time: 10 minutes | **Cooking time:** 30 minutes | **Servings:** 2

Ingredients:

- 1 pound chicken thighs, boneless and skinless
- 2 tablespoons ghee, melted
- 4 asparagus spears, trimmed and halved
- A pinch of salt and black pepper
- ½ cup chicken broth
- ½ teaspoon garam masala
- ½ teaspoon turmeric powder
- ½ teaspoon rosemary, dried
- 1 tablespoon chives, chopped

Directions:

1. Heat up a pan with the ghee over medium heat, add the meat and brown for 5 minutes.
2. Add the rest of the ingredients except the asparagus, toss and cook for 20 minutes.
3. Add the asparagus, toss, cook for 5 minutes more, divide everything between plates and serve.

Nutrition:

calories 500, fat 27, fiber 3, carbs 4, protein 47

Rosemary and Paprika Chicken

Prep time: 10 minutes | **Cooking time:** 25 minutes | **Servings:** 2

Ingredients:

- 1 tablespoon olive oil
- 1 pound chicken breast, skinless, boneless and cubed
- 1 tablespoon ghee, melted
- 1 tablespoon rosemary, chopped
- 1 cup cherry tomatoes, halved
- A pinch of salt and black pepper
- 1 teaspoon sweet paprika

Directions:

1. Heat up a pan with the oil and the ghee over medium heat, add the chicken and brown for 5 minutes.
2. Add the rest of the ingredients, toss, cook for 20 minutes more, divide between plates and serve.

Nutrition:

calories 150, fat 4, fiber 1, carbs 3, protein 10

Poultry Bake

Prep time: 10 minutes | **Cooking time:** 40 minutes | **Servings:** 2

Ingredients:

- 1 pound turkey breast, skinless, boneless and sliced
- 1 tablespoon olive oil
- ½ teaspoon coriander, ground
- ½ teaspoon chili powder
- 1 cup tomato passata (unsweetened)
- 1 teaspoon oregano, dried
- 1 cup mozzarella, sliced
- 1 tablespoon cilantro, chopped

Directions:

1. Grease a baking dish with the oil, arrange the turkey slices inside, add the other ingredients except the cheese and toss.
2. Bake at 390 degrees F for 30 minutes, sprinkle the cheese, cook for 10 minutes more, divide everything between plates and serve.

Nutrition:

calories 320, fat 10, fiber 6, carbs 3, protein 27

Greens and Turkey Bowl

Prep time: 10 minutes | **Cooking time:** 25 minutes | **Servings:** 2

Ingredients:

- 1 cup collard greens, torn
- 1 pound turkey breast, skinless, boneless and cubed
- 2 tablespoons ghee, melted
- 2 garlic cloves, minced
- ½ cup chicken broth
- 1 tablespoon cilantro, chopped
- A pinch of salt and black pepper

Directions:

1. Heat up a pan with the ghee over medium heat, add the garlic and the meat and brown for 5 minutes.
2. Add the rest of the ingredients, toss, cook for 20 minutes more, divide into bowls and serve.

Nutrition:

calories 240, fat 15, fiber 1, carbs 3, protein 25

Tender Turkey in Sauce

Prep time: 10 minutes | **Cooking time:** 30 minutes | **Servings:** 2

Ingredients:

- 1 pound turkey breast, skinless, boneless and cubed
- 2 tablespoons ghee, melted
- 1 tablespoon lime juice
- 1 cup black olives, pitted and chopped
- ¼ cup chicken broth
- A pinch of salt and black pepper
- 1 tablespoon chives, chopped

Directions:

1. Heat up a pan with the ghee over medium heat, add the meat and brown for 5 minutes.
2. Add the rest of the ingredients, toss, cook for 25 minutes, divide between plates and serve.

Nutrition:

calories 384, fat 31, fiber 2, carbs 1, protein 33

Lime Zest Chicken

Prep time: 10 minutes | **Cooking time:** 25 minutes | **Servings:** 2

Ingredients:

- 1 pound chicken thighs, boneless and skinless
- 1 tablespoon olive oil
- 1 tablespoon lime juice
- 1 tablespoon lime zest, grated
- ½ teaspoon turmeric powder
- A pinch of salt and black pepper
- 1 tablespoon chives, chopped

Directions:

1. In a roasting pan, combine the chicken thighs with the oil, lime juice and the other ingredients, toss and cook at 400 degrees F for 25 minutes.
2. Divide the mix between plates and serve.

Nutrition:

calories 495, fat 23.9, fiber 0.5, carbs 0.9, protein 65.8

Chili Powder Turkey

Prep time: 10 minutes | **Cooking time:** 25 minutes | **Servings:** 2

Ingredients:

- 1 pound turkey breast, skinless, boneless and cubed
- 1 tablespoon sage, chopped
- 2 tablespoons olive oil
- ½ cup chicken broth
- ½ teaspoon coriander, ground
- ½ teaspoon chili powder
- A pinch of salt and black pepper
- 1 tablespoon chives, chopped

Directions:

1. Heat up a pan with the oil over medium heat, add the meat and brown for 5 minutes.
2. Add the sage and the other ingredients, toss, cook for 20 minutes more, divide between plates and serve.

Nutrition:

calories 182, fat 9.1, fiber 0.6, carbs 5.2, protein 19.6

Fragrant Cumin Turkey

Prep time: 10 minutes | **Cooking time:** 30 minutes | **Servings:** 2

Ingredients:

- 1 tablespoon ghee, melted
- 1 pound turkey breast, skinless, boneless and cubed
- 1 cup chicken stock
- 1 teaspoon turmeric powder
- ½ teaspoon cumin, ground
- ½ teaspoon coriander, ground
- A pinch of salt and black pepper

Directions:

1. Heat up a pan with the ghee over medium heat, add the chicken and brown for 5 minutes.
2. Add the turmeric and other ingredients, toss, cook for 25 minutes more, divide between plates and serve.

Nutrition:

calories 700, fat 45, fiber 4, carbs 5, protein 45

Poultry and Spinach Mix

Prep time: 10 minutes | **Cooking time:** 30 minutes | **Servings:** 2

Ingredients:

- 1 pound turkey breast, skinless, boneless and sliced
- 1 cup baby spinach
- ¼ cup almonds, chopped
- 1 tablespoon olive oil
- ½ cup chicken broth
- A pinch of salt and black pepper
- ¼ teaspoon coriander, ground
- ½ teaspoon sweet paprika

Directions:

1. In a roasting pan, combine the turkey with the almonds, spinach and the other ingredients, toss and bake at 390 degrees F for 30 minutes.
2. Divide everything between plates and serve.

Nutrition:

calories 320, fat 12, fiber 4, carbs 1, protein 30

Salsa Verde Turkey

Prep time: 10 minutes | **Cooking time:** 30 minutes | **Servings:** 2

Ingredients:

- 1 pound turkey breast, skinless, boneless and cubed
- 1 cup salsa Verde
- 2 shallots, chopped
- 1 tablespoon ghee, melted
- A pinch of salt and black pepper
- 1 teaspoon chili powder
- 1 tablespoon cilantro, chopped

Directions:

1. Heat up a pan with the ghee over medium heat, add the shallots and the meat and brown for 5 minutes.
2. Add the salsa and the other ingredients, toss, cook for 25 minutes more, divide between plates and serve.

Nutrition:

calories 154, fat 5, fiber 3, carbs 2, protein 27

Cilantro Chicken

Prep time: 10 minutes | **Cooking time:** 20 minutes | **Servings:** 2

Ingredients:

- 1 pound chicken thighs, boneless and skinless
- 1 tablespoon ghee, melted
- 4 garlic cloves, minced
- 1 tablespoon olive oil
- ¼ cup cilantro, chopped
- A pinch of salt and black pepper

Directions:

1. Heat up a pan with the ghee and the oil over medium heat, add the garlic and cook for 2 minutes.
2. Add the chicken and the other ingredients, toss, introduce in the oven and cook at 390 degrees F for 18 minutes.
3. Divide everything between plates and serve.

Nutrition:

calories 557, fat 30.3, fiber 0.1, carbs 2.1, protein 66.1

Chicken with Artichokes

Prep time: 10 minutes | **Cooking time:** 25 minutes | **Servings:** 2

Ingredients:

- 2 tablespoons olive oil
- 1 pound chicken breast, skinless, boneless and sliced
- 2 artichokes, trimmed and quartered
- ½ teaspoon chili powder
- A pinch of salt and black pepper
- ½ teaspoon red chili flakes

Directions:

1. In a roasting pan, combine the chicken with the oil, artichokes and the other ingredients, toss and bake at 390 degrees F for 25 minutes.
2. Divide everything between plates and serve.

Nutrition:

calories 457, fat 20, fiber 9, carbs 17.2, protein 53.5

Hot Chicken

Prep time: 10 minutes | **Cooking time:** 25 minutes | **Servings:** 2

Ingredients:

- 1 pound chicken breast, skinless, boneless and cubed
- 1 tablespoon ghee, melted
- ¼ cup chicken broth
- 1 teaspoon turmeric powder
- 1 teaspoon sweet paprika
- ¼ cup jalapenos, chopped
- A pinch of salt and black pepper
- 1 tablespoon chives, chopped

Directions:

1. Heat up a pan with the ghee over medium heat, add the jalapenos and cook for 5 minutes.
2. Add the meat and brown for 5 minutes more.
3. Add the rest of the ingredients, toss, cook for 15 minutes more, divide between plates and serve.

Nutrition:

calories 340, fat 12, fiber 2, carbs 5, protein 20

Chicken and Leek Bowl

Prep time: 10 minutes | **Cooking time:** 30 minutes | **Servings:** 2

Ingredients:

- 1 pound chicken breast, skinless, boneless and sliced
- 1 tablespoon ghee, melted
- ½ cup kalamata olives, pitted and halved
- 2 leeks, sliced
- ½ teaspoon chili powder
- ½ teaspoon hot paprika
- ½ cup chicken broth
- A pinch of salt and black pepper
- 1 tablespoon cilantro, chopped

Directions:

1. In a roasting pan, combine the chicken with the ghee, olives and the other ingredients, toss, and bake at 390 degrees F for 30 minutes.
2. Divide everything between plates and serve.

Nutrition:

calories 267, fat 5.6, fiber 0, carbs 6.0, protein 35

Thyme Chicken

Prep time: 10 minutes | **Cooking time:** 25 minutes | **Servings:** 2

Ingredients:

- 2 garlic cloves, minced
- 1 tablespoon olive oil
- 1 pound chicken breast, skinless, boneless and cubed
- ¼ cup coconut, unsweetened and shredded
- ¼ cup chicken broth
- ¼ cup coconut milk
- 1 teaspoon thyme, dried
- 1 tablespoon parsley, chopped
- A pinch of salt and black pepper

Directions:

1. Heat up a pan with the oil over medium heat, add the garlic and the chicken and brown for 5 minutes.
2. Add the rest of the ingredients, toss, cook for 20 minutes more, divide between plates and serve.

Nutrition:

calories 364, fat 22, fiber 2, carbs 4, protein 24

Tender Duck

Prep time: 10 minutes | **Cooking time:** 30 minutes | **Servings:** 2

Ingredients:

- 1 pound duck breasts, skinless, boneless and cubed
- 2 red chilies, minced
- ½ teaspoon chili powder
- ¼ cup chicken broth
- 1 tablespoon ghee, melted
- 2 shallots, chopped
- A pinch of salt and black pepper

Directions:

1. Heat up a pan with the ghee over medium heat, add the meat and brown for 5 minutes.
2. Add the rest of the ingredients, toss, cook for 25 minutes more, divide between plates and serve.

Nutrition:

calories 450, fat 23, fiber 3, carbs 8.3, protein 50

Mustard Powder Turkey

Prep time: 10 minutes | **Cooking time:** 30 minutes | **Servings:** 2

Ingredients:

- 1 pound turkey breast, skinless, boneless and sliced
- 2 tablespoons olive oil
- 1 tablespoon thyme, chopped
- 1 tablespoon basil, chopped
- 2 garlic cloves, minced
- 1 teaspoon mustard powder
- 1 teaspoon cayenne powder
- A pinch of salt and black pepper
- ¼ cup chicken broth

Directions:

1. In a roasting pan, combine the turkey with the oil, thyme and the other ingredients, toss and cook at 390 degrees F for 30 minutes.
2. Divide the turkey mix between plates and serve.

Nutrition:

calories 360, fat 23, fiber 2, carbs 6, protein 23

Chili Chicken Wings

Prep time: 5 minutes | **Cooking time:** 25 minutes | **Servings:** 2

Ingredients:

- 1 pound chicken wings
- 1 tablespoon ghee, melted
- 1 tablespoons coriander, chopped
- 1 teaspoon chili powder
- A pinch of salt and black pepper
- 1 teaspoon sweet paprika

Directions:

1. Heat up a pan with the ghee over medium heat, add the chicken wings and brown them for 2 minutes on each side.
2. Add the rest of the ingredients, toss, introduce in the oven and cook at 390 degrees F for 20 minutes more.
3. Divide everything between plates and serve with a side salad.

Nutrition:

calories 494, fat 23.4, fiber 0.9, carbs 1.4, protein 66

Ketogenic Meat Recipes

Pork and Zucchini

Prep time: 10 minutes | **Cooking time:** 30 minutes | **Servings:** 2

Ingredients:

- 2 garlic cloves, minced
- 1 pound pork stew meat, cubed
- 1 tablespoon olive oil
- 2 zucchinis, cubed
- 2 shallots, chopped
- ½ cup beef stock
- A pinch of salt and black pepper
- 1 teaspoon cumin, ground

Directions:

1. Heat up a pan with the oil over medium heat, add the shallots and the garlic and cook for 5 minutes.
2. Add the meat and brown for 5 minutes more.
3. Add the rest of the ingredients, toss, cook for 20 minutes more, divide everything between plates and serve.

Nutrition:

calories 222, fat 10, fiber 2, carbs 8, protein 21

Parmesan Meat

Prep time: 10 minutes | **Cooking time:** 30 minutes | **Servings:** 2

Ingredients:

- 1 pound beef stew meat, ground
- ¼ cup beef stock
- 2 tablespoons ghee, melted
- ¼ cup parmesan, grated
- 3 scallions, chopped
- ½ teaspoon sweet paprika
- ½ teaspoon rosemary, dried
- A pinch of salt and black pepper
- ½ teaspoon red pepper flakes, crushed
- A pinch of cayenne pepper

Directions:

1. Heat up a pan with the ghee over medium heat, add the scallions and the meat and brown for 5 minutes.
2. Add the rest of the ingredients except the parmesan, and toss.
3. Sprinkle the parmesan on top and cook the mix for 25 minutes more, stirring often.
4. Divide everything between plates and serve.

Nutrition:

calories 456, fat 35, fiber 3, carbs 4, protein 32

Tender Lamb with Ghee

Prep time: 10 minutes | **Cooking time:** 30 minutes | **Servings:** 2

Ingredients:

- 1 pound lamb stew meat, cubed
- 2 leeks, sliced
- ½ teaspoon rosemary, dried
- 1 teaspoon chili powder
- 2 tablespoons ghee, melted
- A pinch of salt and black pepper
- 1 cup beef stock
- 1 tablespoon cilantro, chopped

Directions:

1. Heat up a pan with the ghee over medium heat, add the leeks and sauté for 5 minutes.
2. Add the meat and brown for 5 minutes more.
3. Add the rest of the ingredients, toss, cook for 20 minutes more, divide between plates and serve.

Nutrition:

calories 260, fat 7, fiber 2, carbs 4, protein 10

Cheesy Cumin and Garlic Beef

Prep time: 10 minutes | **Cooking time:** 30 minutes | **Servings:** 2

Ingredients:

- 1 pound beef stew meat, cubed
- 1 tablespoon olive oil
- 3 scallions, chopped
- ½ teaspoon sweet paprika
- ½ teaspoon cumin, ground
- 2 garlic cloves, minced
- A pinch of salt and black pepper
- 1 cup mozzarella cheese, shredded
- ½ cup beef stock
- 1 tablespoon chives, chopped

Directions:

1. Heat up a pan with the oil over medium heat, add the scallions and garlic and cook for 5 minutes.
2. Add the meat and brown for 5 minutes more.
3. Add the rest of the ingredients except the mozzarella, toss and cook for 15 minutes more.
4. Sprinkle the cheese on top, introduce the pan in the oven and cook at 390 degrees F for 5 minutes more.
5. Divide everything between plates and serve.

Nutrition:

calories 554, fat 51, fiber 3, carbs 5, protein 45

Autumn Beef Mix

Prep time: 10 minutes | **Cooking time:** 30 minutes | **Servings:** 2

Ingredients:

- 1 pound beef stew meat, cubed
- 1 tablespoon olive oil
- 3 scallions, chopped
- 1 teaspoon cinnamon powder
- ½ teaspoon cumin, ground
- ½ teaspoon coriander, ground
- 2 garlic cloves, minced
- 1 cup beef stock
- ½ teaspoon sweet paprika
- 1 tablespoon cilantro, chopped
- A pinch of salt and black pepper

Directions:

1. Heat up a pan with oil over medium heat, add the scallions and the garlic and cook for 5 minutes.
2. Add the meat and cook for 5 minutes more.
3. Add the rest of the ingredients, toss, cook for 20 minutes more, divide between plates and serve.

Nutrition:

calories 320, fat 13, fiber 4, carbs 12, protein 40

Nutmeg Pork Cubes

Prep time: 10 minutes | **Cooking time:** 30 minutes | **Servings:** 2

Ingredients:

- 1 pound pork stew meat, cubed
- ½ cup beef stock
- 1 tablespoon avocado oil
- ½ teaspoon allspice, ground
- ½ teaspoon onion powder
- ½ teaspoon turmeric powder
- ¼ teaspoon nutmeg, ground
- A pinch of salt and black pepper
- 1 teaspoon garlic powder
- 1 tablespoon chives, chopped

Directions:

1. Heat up a pan with the oil over medium heat, add the meat and brown for 5 minutes.
2. Add the stock and the rest of the ingredients, toss, cook for 25 minutes more, divide between plates and serve with a side salad.

Nutrition:

calories 267, fat 23, fiber 1, carbs 3, protein 12

Beef and Peppers

Prep time: 10 minutes | **Cooking time:** 35 minutes | **Servings:** 2

Ingredients:

- 1 pound beef stew meat
- 1 tablespoon capers, drained
- 1 cup baby kale
- 2 tablespoons avocado oil
- 1 red bell pepper, chopped
- 1 red chili pepper, minced
- 1 cup tomato passata (unsweetened)
- 2 tablespoons cilantro, chopped
- A pinch of salt and black pepper
- 1 teaspoon cumin, ground
- 1 tablespoon cilantro, chopped
- 1 teaspoon oregano, dried

Directions:

1. Heat up a pan with the oil over medium heat, add the bell pepper and chili pepper and cook for 5 minutes.
2. Add the meat and brown for 5 minutes more.
3. Add the rest of the ingredients, toss, cook for 25 minutes, divide between plates and serve.

Nutrition:

calories 305, fat 14, fiber 4, carbs 8, protein 25

Pork and Cauli Mix

Prep time: 10 minutes | **Cooking time:** 40 minutes | **Servings:** 2

Ingredients:

- 1 pound pork stew meat cubed
- 1 tablespoon olive oil
- 1 cup cauliflower florets
- ½ teaspoon cumin, ground
- ½ teaspoon rosemary, dried
- ½ teaspoon sweet paprika
- 1 cup tomato passata (unsweetened)
- A pinch of salt and black pepper

Directions:

1. Heat up a pan with the oil over medium heat, add the meat and brown for 5 minutes.
2. Add the cauliflower and the other ingredients, toss, cook for 35 minutes more, divide between plates and serve.

Nutrition:

calories 320, fat 20, fiber 3, carbs 6, protein 23

Coriander Meat Stew

Prep time: 10 minutes | **Cooking time:** 1 hour

Servings: 2

Ingredients:

- 1 pound lamb stew meat, cubed
- 2 tablespoons ghee, melted
- 3 scallions, chopped
- 2 garlic cloves, minced
- 1 cup mushrooms, halved
- 1 cup cherry tomatoes, halved
- 1 cup tomato passata (unsweetened)
- 1 teaspoon coriander, ground
- 1 teaspoon rosemary, dried
- 1 tablespoon cilantro, chopped
- A pinch of salt and black pepper
- 1 cup water

Directions:

1. Heat up a pot with the ghee over medium heat, add the scallions and the garlic and cook for 5 minutes.
2. Add the mushrooms and cook for another 5 minutes.
3. Add the meat and cook for 5 minutes.
4. Add the rest of the ingredients, toss, bring to a simmer and cook for 45 minutes.
5. Divide into bowls and serve.

Nutrition:

calories 254, fat 15, fiber 1, carbs 3, protein 23

Juicy Rosemary Pork

Prep time: 10 minutes | **Cooking time:** 35 minutes

Servings: 2

Ingredients:

- 1 pound pork loin, cubed
- 1 tablespoon avocado oil
- 1 teaspoon sweet paprika
- ½ teaspoon rosemary, dried
- A pinch of salt and black pepper
- 2 scallions, chopped
- 2 garlic cloves, minced
- 1 tablespoon lime juice
- 1 tablespoon cilantro, chopped

Directions:

1. Heat up a pan with the oil over medium heat, add the scallions and garlic and cook for 5 minutes.
2. Add the meat and brown for 5 minutes more.
3. Add the rest of the ingredients, toss, cook for 25 minutes more, divide everything between plates and serve.

Nutrition:

calories 572, fat 32.7, fiber 1.4, carbs 3.3, protein 62.7

Garlic Mushroom with Bok Choy

Prep time: 10 minutes | **Cooking time:** 20 minutes | **Servings:** 2

Ingredients:

- 1 cup mushrooms, halved
- 2 tablespoons ghee, melted
- 2 scallions, chopped
- 2 garlic cloves, minced
- ½ teaspoon turmeric powder
- A pinch of salt and black pepper
- 1 bunch bok choy, chopped
- ½ teaspoon red pepper flakes
- 1 tablespoon balsamic vinegar
- 1 tablespoon chives, chopped

Directions:

1. Heat up a pan with the ghee over medium heat, add the scallions and garlic and cook for 5 minutes.
2. Add the mushrooms, stir and cook for 5 minutes more.
3. Add the bok choy and the other ingredients, toss, cook for 10 minutes, divide into bowls and serve.

Nutrition:

calories 100, fat 3, fiber 1, carbs 2, protein 6

Chives and Avocado Mix

Prep time: 10 minutes | **Cooking time:** 15 minutes

Servings: 2

Ingredients:

- 2 garlic cloves, minced
- 2 cup bok choy, chopped
- 1 avocado, peeled, pitted and cubed
- 1 tablespoon olive oil
- 2 scallions, chopped
- ½ cup tomato passata (unsweetened)
- 1 tablespoon chives, chopped
- A pinch of salt and black pepper

Directions:

1. Heat up a pan with the oil over medium heat, add the garlic and the scallions, stir and cook for 2 minutes.
2. Add the bok choy and the other ingredients, toss, cook for 13 minutes more, divide into bowls and serve.

Nutrition:

calories 50, fat 1, fiber 1, carbs 2, protein 2

Spring Pork Stew

Prep time: 10 minutes | Cooking time: 1 hour | Servings: 2

Ingredients:

- 1 pound pork stew meat, cubed
- 1 tablespoon avocado oil
- 3 scallions, chopped
- 2 garlic cloves, minced
- 1 cup cherry tomatoes, halved
- 1 zucchini, cubed
- A pinch of salt and black pepper
- 1 cup tomato passata (unsweetened)
- ¼ cup beef stock
- ½ teaspoon coriander, ground
- ½ teaspoon sweet paprika
- 1 tablespoon cilantro, chopped

Directions:

1. Heat up a pot with the oil over medium heat, add the scallions and the garlic and cook for 5 minutes.
2. Add the meat and brown for 5 more minutes.
3. Add the rest of the ingredients, toss, bring to a simmer and cook for 50 minutes more, stirring often.
4. Divide the stew into bowls and serve.

Nutrition:

calories 400, fat 25, fiber 3, carbs 6, protein 43

Spicy Okra and Beef Bowl

Prep time: 10 minutes | Cooking time: 30 minutes | Servings: 2

Ingredients:

- 1 pound beef stew meat, cubed
- 2 scallions, chopped
- 2 garlic cloves, minced
- 1 tablespoon avocado oil
- 1 green bell pepper, chopped
- A pinch of salt and black pepper
- 1 cup tomato passata (unsweetened)
- ½ cup beef stock
- ½ teaspoon chili powder
- 1 cup okra, sliced
- 1 tablespoon parsley, chopped

Directions:

1. Heat up a pot with the oil over medium heat, add the scallions and the garlic and cook for 5 minutes.
2. Add the meat and brown for 5 minutes more.
3. Add the rest of the ingredients, bring to a simmer and cook everything for 20 minutes stirring often, divide into bowls and serve.

Nutrition:

calories 274, fat 20, fiber 4, carbs 7, protein 10

Keto Meat with Vegetables

Prep time: 10 minutes | Cooking time: 35 minutes | Servings: 2

Ingredients:

- 1 pound beef stew meat
- 2 tablespoons ghee, melted
- 2 scallions, chopped
- 1 cup okra, sliced
- 1 cup mushrooms, halved
- 1 cup beef stock
- ½ teaspoon sweet paprika
- ½ teaspoon coriander, ground
- ½ teaspoon rosemary, dried
- A pinch of salt and black pepper
- 1 tablespoon cilantro, chopped

Directions:

1. Heat up a pan with the ghee over medium heat, add the scallions and the meat and brown for 5 minutes.
2. Add the mushrooms and cook them for another 5 minutes.
3. Add the rest of the ingredients, toss, cook for 25 minutes more, divide into bowls and serve.

Nutrition:

calories 275, fat 13, fiber 4, carbs 7, protein 28

Pork with Coriander and Shredded Cabbage

Prep time: 10 minutes | Cooking time: 30 minutes | Servings: 2

Ingredients:

- 1 tablespoon olive oil
- 1 pound pork stew meat, cubed
- 1 cup cherry tomatoes, halved
- 1 cup green cabbage, shredded
- ½ teaspoon sweet paprika
- ½ teaspoon coriander, ground
- A pinch of salt and black pepper
- 1 cup beef stock
- 2 tablespoons parsley, chopped

Directions:

1. Heat up a pan with the oil over medium heat, add the meat and brown for 5 minutes.
2. Add the cabbage and cook for 5 minutes more.
3. Add the rest of the ingredients, toss, cook for 20 minutes more, divide into bowls and serve.

Nutrition:

calories 200, fat 12, fiber 2, carbs 6, protein 15

Aromatic Parsley and Lamb Stew

Prep time: 10 minutes | Cooking time: 40 minutes | Servings: 2

Ingredients:

- 1 pound lamb stew meat, cubed
- 1 cup okra, sliced
- 3 scallions, chopped
- 2 garlic cloves, minced
- 1 tablespoon olive oil
- 1 cup beef stock
- A pinch of salt and black pepper
- 1 orange bell pepper, chopped
- 1 red bell pepper, chopped
- A pinch of red pepper flakes
- 1 tablespoon parsley, chopped

Directions:

1. Heat up a pan with the oil over medium heat, add the scallions and the garlic and cook for 5 minutes.
2. Add the meat and brown for 5 minutes more.
3. Add the rest of the ingredients, toss, bring to a simmer and cook for 30 minutes.
4. Divide into bowls and serve.

Nutrition:

calories 200, fat 5, fiber 3, carbs 6, protein 14

Cumin and Bell Pepper Pork

Prep time: 10 minutes | Cooking time: 35 minutes | Servings: 2

Ingredients:

- 1 cup beef stock
- 1 tablespoon olive oil
- 1 teaspoon cumin, ground
- 1 tablespoon cilantro, chopped
- 2 garlic cloves, minced
- 1 pound pork stew meat, cubed
- 1 green bell pepper, cut into strips
- 1 red bell pepper, cut into strips
- 1 yellow bell pepper, cut into strips
- A pinch of salt and black pepper

Directions:

1. Heat up a pan with the oil over medium heat, add the garlic and the peppers and cook for 5 minutes.
2. Add the meat and cook for 5 minutes more.
3. Add the rest of the ingredients, toss, cook for 25 minutes, divide everything into bowls and serve.

Nutrition:

calories 224, fat 15, fiber 1, carbs 3, protein 19

Chives Radishes

Prep time: 10 minutes | **Cooking time:** 25 minutes | **Servings:** 2

Ingredients:
- 1 tablespoon avocado oil
- ½ pound radishes, halved
- 1 tablespoon chives, chopped
- 2 tablespoons lime juice
- ½ teaspoon garam masala
- A pinch of salt and black pepper

Directions:
1. Spread the radishes on a baking sheet lined with parchment paper, add the oil and the other ingredients, toss and cook at 380 degrees F for 25 minutes.
2. Divide the radishes between plates and serve.

Nutrition:
calories 160, fat 7, fiber 2, carbs 6, protein 10

Rosemary Tomatoes

Prep time: 10 minutes | **Cooking time:** 20 minutes | **Servings:** 2

Ingredients:
- ¼ cup shallots, chopped
- 1 tablespoon olive oil
- ½ pound cherry tomatoes, halved
- ½ teaspoon sweet paprika
- A pinch of salt and black pepper
- 1 teaspoon rosemary, dried

Directions:
1. In a roasting pan, combine the tomatoes with the shallots and the tomatoes and the other ingredients, toss and bake at 390 degrees F for 20 minutes.
2. Divide between plates and serve.

Nutrition:
calories 200, fat 12, fiber 2, carbs 5, protein 14

Chili Fennel

Prep time: 10 minutes | **Cooking time:** 20 minutes | **Servings:** 2

Ingredients:
- 2 fennel bulbs, sliced
- 2 tablespoons ghee, melted
- 1 tablespoon lime juice
- A pinch of salt and black pepper
- 1 teaspoon cumin, ground
- ½ teaspoon rosemary, dried
- 1 teaspoon chili powder

Directions:
1. In a roasting pan, combine the fennel with the ghee and the other ingredients, toss and cook at 390 degrees F for 20 minutes.
2. Divide everything between plates and serve.

Nutrition:
calories 256, fat 23, fiber 2, carbs 5, protein 13

Garlic and Chives Asparagus

Prep time: 10 minutes | **Cooking time:** 12 minutes | **Servings:** 2

Ingredients:
- ½ pound asparagus spears, trimmed
- 1 tablespoon avocado oil
- 2 garlic cloves, minced
- ½ teaspoon chili powder
- ½ teaspoon sweet paprika
- A pinch of salt and black pepper
- 1 tablespoon chives, chopped

Directions:
1. In a roasting pan, combine the asparagus with the oil, garlic and the other ingredients, toss and cook at 380 degrees F for 12 minutes.
2. Divide everything between plates and serve.

Nutrition:
calories 100, fat 3, fiber 1, carbs 2, protein 6

Olives and Scallions Salad

Prep time: 10 minutes | **Servings:** 2

Ingredients:
- 2 cucumbers, sliced
- ½ cup kalamata olives, pitted and halved
- 1 tablespoon chives, chopped
- 2 tablespoons olive oil
- 2 scallions, chopped
- 2 tablespoons lemon juice
- Salt and black pepper to the taste

Directions:
1. In a bowl, combine the cucumbers with the olives and the other ingredients, toss and serve.

Nutrition:
calories 140, fat 4, fiber 2, carbs 4, protein 5

Spring Salad

Prep time: 10 minutes | **Servings:** 2

Ingredients:
- 2 cups cherry tomatoes, halved
- 1 tablespoon olive oil
- 2 scallions, chopped
- 1 teaspoon sweet paprika
- 1 tablespoon lemon juice
- ½ cup black olives, pitted and halved
- A pinch of salt and black pepper

Directions:
1. In a bowl, combine the tomatoes with the olives, scallions and the other ingredients, toss and serve.

Nutrition:
calories 332, fat 23, fiber 4, carbs 6, protein 6

Baby Kale Mix

Prep time: 10 minutes | **Cooking time:** 15 minutes | **Servings:** 2

Ingredients:
- 1 cup baby spinach
- 1 cup baby kale
- 2 tablespoons ghee, melted
- 2 scallions, chopped
- ½ teaspoon sweet paprika
- ½ cup tomato passata (unsweetened)
- 1/3 cup cilantro, chopped
- A pinch of salt and black pepper

Directions:
1. Heat up a pan with the ghee over medium heat, add the scallions and the paprika and cook for 2 minutes.
2. Add the spinach and the other ingredients, toss, cook for 13 minutes more, divide between plates and serve.

Nutrition:
calories 300, fat 23, fiber 5, carbs 6, protein 17

Cilantro Avocado

Prep time: 10 minutes | **Servings:** 2

Ingredients:
- 2 avocados, peeled, pitted and roughly cubed
- 1 tablespoon cilantro, chopped
- Juice of 1 lime
- Zest of 1 lime, grated
- 1 cup cherry tomatoes, halved
- A pinch of salt and black pepper

Directions:
1. In a bowl, combine the avocados with the tomatoes and the other ingredients, toss and serve.

Nutrition:
calories 240, fat 4, fiber 2, carbs 6, protein 12

Cherry Tomatoes and Greens Salad

Prep time: 10 minutes | **Servings:** 2

Ingredients:

- 2 cups baby arugula
- 1 cup cherry tomatoes, halved
- 1 tablespoon avocado oil
- 2 tablespoons walnuts, chopped
- 2 tablespoons cilantro, chopped
- Salt and black pepper to the taste
- 1 tablespoon lemon juice

Directions:

1. In a bowl, combine the cherry tomatoes with the arugula and the other ingredients, toss and serve.

Nutrition:

calories 200, fat 2, fiber 1, carbs 5, protein 7

Paprika and Lime Bok Choy

Prep time: 10 minutes | **Cooking time:** 15 minutes | **Servings:** 2

Ingredients:

- 1 tablespoon olive oil
- 2 garlic cloves, minced
- 2 cups bok choy, torn
- 1 tablespoon lime juice
- 2 tablespoons chives, chopped
- ½ teaspoon sweet paprika
- ½ cup coconut cream
- Salt and black pepper to the taste

Directions:

1. Heat up a pan with the oil over medium heat, add the garlic and cook for 3 minutes.
2. Add the bok choy and the other ingredients, toss, cook for 12 minutes more, divide between plates and serve.

Nutrition:

calories 200, fat 4, fiber 2, carbs 6, protcin 10

Broccoli Florets Bowl

Prep time: 10 minutes | **Cooking time:** 20 minutes | **Servings:** 2

Ingredients:

- 2 scallions, chopped
- 1 cup baby spinach
- 1 cup broccoli florets
- 1 teaspoon chili powder
- ½ cup veggie stock
- 1 tablespoon olive oil
- 1 garlic clove, minced
- A pinch of salt and black pepper
- 1 tablespoon dill, chopped

Directions:

1. Heat up a pan with the oil over medium heat, add the scallions and chili powder and cook for 5 minutes.
2. Add the spinach, broccoli and the other ingredients, toss, cook for 15 minutes more, divide between plates and serve.

Nutrition:

calories 150, fat 3, fiber 1, carbs 3, protein 7

Zucchini Cubes Stew

Prep time: 10 minutes | **Cooking time:** 20 minutes | **Servings:** 2

Ingredients:

- 2 zucchinis, roughly cubed
- 1 tablespoon ghee, melted
- 3 scallions, chopped
- 2 garlic cloves, minced
- ½ teaspoon rosemary, dried
- ¼ cup veggie stock
- 1 tablespoon dill, chopped

Directions:

1. Heat up a pan with the ghee over medium heat, add the scallions and the garlic and cook for 5 minutes.
2. Add the zucchinis and the other ingredients, toss, cook for 15 minutes more, divide everything between plates and serve.

Nutrition:

calories 160, fat 4, fiber 2, carbs 4, protein 8

Asparagus Stew

Prep time: 10 minutes | **Cooking time:** 10 minutes | **Servings:** 2

Ingredients:

- 1 asparagus bunch, trimmed and halved
- 2 tablespoons ghee, melted
- Zest of ½ lemon, grated
- 1 tablespoon lemon juice
- ¼ cup veggie stock
- A pinch of salt and black pepper
- 1 tablespoon chives, chopped

Directions:

1. Heat up a pan with the ghee over medium heat, add the asparagus, lemon juice and the other ingredients, toss, cook for 10 minutes, divide between plates and serve.

Nutrition:

calories 130, fat 1, fiber 1, carbs 2, protein 3

Cheesy Artichokes

Prep time: 10 minutes | **Cooking time:** 20 minutes | **Servings:** 2

Ingredients:

- ¼ cup parmesan, grated
- 2 artichokes, trimmed and halved
- 1 tablespoon ghee, melted
- 1 tablespoon lime juice
- A pinch of salt and black pepper
- ½ teaspoon turmeric powder
- 1 tablespoon rosemary, chopped

Directions:

1. In a roasting pan, combine the artichokes with the ghee and the other ingredients except the parmesan and toss.
2. Sprinkle the parmesan on top, bake at 390 degrees F for 20 minutes, divide between plates and serve.

Nutrition:

calories 120, fat 2, fiber 2, carbs 5, protein 8

Basil Green Beans

Prep time: 10 minutes | **Cooking time:** 20 minutes | **Servings:** 2

Ingredients:

- ½ pound green beans, trimmed and halved
- A pinch of salt and black pepper
- 2 tablespoons ghee, melted
- 1 teaspoon basil, dried
- 1 tablespoon chives, chopped

Directions:

1. In a roasting pan combine the green beans with the ghee and the other ingredients, toss and cook at 380 degrees F fro 20 minutes.
2. Divide between plates and serve.

Nutrition:

calories 122, fat 12, fiber 1, carbs 3, protein 14

Sprouts and Kale Bowl

Prep time: 10 minutes | **Cooking time:** 20 minutes | **Servings:** 2

Ingredients:

- 1 tablespoon ghee, melted
- ½ pound Brussels sprouts, trimmed and halved
- 1 cup baby kale
- ½ teaspoon garam masala
- ½ teaspoon sweet paprika
- A pinch of salt and black pepper
- 1 tablespoon lime juice

Directions:

1. In a roasting pan, combine the sprouts with the kale and the other ingredients, toss and cook at 390 degrees F for 20 minutes.
2. Divide everything between plates and serve.

Nutrition:

calories 80, fat 5, fiber 2, carbs 5, protein 7

Greens Bowl

Prep time: 10 minutes | **Cooking time:** 15 minutes | **Servings:** 2

Ingredients:

- 1 tablespoon olive oil
- 1 pound baby spinach
- 3 scallions, chopped
- 2 garlic cloves, minced
- ½ cup veggie stock
- ½ teaspoon coriander, ground
- A pinch of salt and black pepper
- 1 tablespoon cilantro, chopped

Directions:

1. Heat up a pan with the oil over medium heat, add the garlic and the scallions and cook for 2 minutes.
2. Add the spinach and the other ingredients, toss, cook for 13 minutes more, divide into bowls and serve.

Nutrition:

calories 143, fat 6, fiber 3, carbs 7, protein 7

Coconut Cream Bok Choy

Prep time: 10 minutes | **Cooking time:** 20 minutes | **Servings:** 2

Ingredients:

- ½ pound bok choy, torn
- 2 scallions, chopped
- 1 tablespoon olive oil
- 1 cup coconut cream
- Salt and black pepper to the taste
- 1 tablespoon cilantro, chopped

Directions:

1. Heat up a pan with the oil over medium heat, add the scallions and cook for 5 minutes.
2. Add the bok choy and the other ingredients, toss, cook for 15 minutes, divide between plates and serve.

Nutrition:

calories 30, fat 1, fiber 0.4, carbs 1, protein 0.1

Black Pepper Radishes

Prep time: 10 minutes | **Cooking time:** 20 minutes | **Servings:** 2

Ingredients:

- ½ pound radishes, halved
- 2 tablespoons ghee, melted
- 1 tablespoon cheddar cheese, grated
- A pinch of red pepper flakes, crushed
- Salt and black pepper to the taste

Directions:

1. Heat up a pan with the ghee over medium heat, add the radishes, pepper flakes, salt and pepper, stir and cook for 15 minutes.
2. Sprinkle the cheese on top, cook for 5 minutes more, divide between plates and serve.

Nutrition:

calories 340, fat 23, fiber 3, carbs 6, protein 15

Baby Kale and Halved Radish

Prep time: 10 minutes | **Cooking time:** 20 minutes | **Servings:** 2

Ingredients:

- ½ pound baby kale
- 1 cup radishes, halved
- 1 tablespoon olive oil
- Juice of 1 lime
- ½ teaspoon turmeric powder
- ½ teaspoon cumin, ground
- ½ cup veggie stock
- 1 tablespoon chives, chopped

Directions:

1. Heat up a pan with the oil over medium heat, add the radishes and cook for 5 minutes.
2. Add the kale and the other ingredients, toss, cook for 15 minutes more, divide between plates and serve.

Nutrition:

calories 120, fat 2, fiber 1, carbs 3, protein 10

Keto Broccoli Mix

Prep time: 10 minutes | **Cooking time:** 20 minutes | **Servings:** 2

Ingredients:

- 2 cups broccoli florets
- 1 tablespoon balsamic vinegar
- 2 scallions, chopped
- 1 tablespoon ghee, melted
- 1 bunch Swiss chard, chopped
- ½ cup veggie stock
- 1 green bell pepper, chopped
- Salt and black pepper to the taste
- 2 teaspoons thyme, chopped
- 1 teaspoon rosemary, dried

Directions:

1. Heat up a pan with the ghee over medium heat, add the scallions and the bell pepper and cook for 5 minutes.
2. Add the rest of the ingredients, toss, cook for 15 minutes more, divide into bowls and serve.

Nutrition:

calories 150, fat 8, fiber 2, carbs 4, protein 9

Basil Cream

Prep time: 10 minutes | **Cooking time:** 45 minutes | **Servings:** 2

Ingredients:

- 1 pound cherry tomatoes, halved
- 4 scallions, chopped
- 1 green chili, minced
- 2 tablespoons olive oil
- 1 tablespoon basil, hopped
- A pinch of salt and black pepper
- 2 cups chicken broth
- 1 tablespoon chives, chopped

Directions:

1. Spread the tomatoes on a baking sheet lined with parchment paper, add the scallions, chili, oil and basil, toss and roast at 400 degrees F for 30 minutes.
2. Heat up a pot with the stock over medium heat, add the roasted tomatoes and the other ingredients, toss, simmer for 15 minutes, blend using an immersion blender, divide into bowls and serve cold.

Nutrition:

calories 140, fat 2, fiber 2, carbs 5, protein 8

Coconut Cream Zucchini

Prep time: 10 minutes | **Cooking time:** 20 minutes | **Servings:** 2

Ingredients:

- 2 zucchinis, roughly cubed
- 1 avocado, peeled, pitted and roughly cubed
- 2 tablespoons ghee, melted
- 3 scallions, minced
- 2 garlic cloves, minced
- ½ teaspoon turmeric powder
- 1 cup coconut cream
- A pinch of salt and black pepper
- 1 tablespoon cilantro, chopped

Directions:

1. Heat up a pan with the ghee over medium heat, add the scallions and garlic and cook for 5 minutes.
2. Add the zucchinis, stir and cook for 10 minutes more.
3. Add the rest of the ingredients, toss, cook for another 5 minutes, divide into bowls and serve.

Nutrition:

calories 180, fat 2, fiber 3, carbs 5, protein 10

Chili and Chives Lamb

Prep time: 10 minutes | **Cooking time:** 30 minutes | **Servings:** 2

Ingredients:
- 2 tablespoons ginger, grated
- 1 pound lamb stew meat, cubed
- 2 scallions, chopped
- ¼ cup beef stock
- 2 garlic cloves, minced
- ½ teaspoon cloves, crushed
- 2 tablespoons ghee, melted
- 1 teaspoon garama masala
- ½ teaspoon chili powder
- 1 tablespoon chives, chopped

Directions:
1. Heat up a pan with the ghee over medium heat, add the ginger, scallions and garlic and cook for 5 minutes.
2. Add the meat and cook for 5 minutes more.
3. Add the rest of the ingredients, toss, cook for 20 minutes, divide into bowls and serve.

Nutrition:
calories 160, fat 6, fiber 3, carbs 7, protein 20

Scallions and Celery Stalk Lamb

Prep time: 10 minutes | **Cooking time:** 30 minutes | **Servings:** 2

Ingredients:
- 1 pound lamb stew meat, cubed
- 2 tablespoons ghee, melted
- 3 scallions, chopped
- 2 garlic cloves, minced
- 1 celery stalks, chopped
- ½ cup beef stock
- ¼ cup tomato passata (unsweetened)
- A pinch of salt and black pepper
- 1 tablespoon chives, chopped

Directions:
1. Heat up a pan with the ghee over medium heat, add the scallions and the garlic and cook for 5 minutes.
2. Add the meat and cook for 5 minutes more.
3. Add the rest of the ingredients, toss, cook for 20 minutes more, divide into bowls and serve.

Nutrition:
calories 700, fat 43, fiber 6, carbs 10, protein 67

Keto Lamb Bowl

Prep time: 10 minutes | **Cooking time:** 40 minutes | **Servings:** 2

Ingredients:
- 2 garlic cloves, minced
- 4 spring onions, chopped
- 2 tablespoons ghee, melted
- 1 tablespoon olive oil
- 1 pound lamb stew meat, cubed
- ½ cup cherry tomatoes, halved
- A pinch of salt and black pepper
- ½ cup beef stock
- 1 tablespoon chives, chopped

Directions:
1. Heat up a pan with the ghee over medium heat, add the spring onions and the garlic and cook for 5 minutes.
2. Add the meat and brown for 5 minutes more.
3. Add the rest of the ingredients, toss, cook for 30 minutes more, divide into bowls and serve.

Nutrition:
calories 324, fat 4, fiber 5, carbs 8, protein 20

Pork Chops with Vegetables

Prep time: 10 minutes | **Cooking time:** 30 minutes | **Servings:** 2

Ingredients:
- 2 pork chops
- 4 asparagus spears, trimmed and halved
- 1 tablespoon olive oil
- 2 shallots, chopped
- 1 tablespoon chives, chopped
- ¼ cup beef stock
- A pinch of salt and black pepper

Directions:
1. Heat up a pan with the oil over medium heat, add the shallots and cook for 2 minutes.
2. Add the meat and brown for 3 minutes more.
3. Add the rest of the ingredients, toss, cook for 25 minutes more, divide between plates and serve.

Nutrition:
calories 328, fat 27, fiber 1.1, carbs 2, protein 19.4

Green Beans with Chili Pork

Prep time: 10 minutes | **Cooking time:** 30 minutes | **Servings:** 2

Ingredients:
- 2 tablespoons olive oil
- 2 pork chops
- 1 cup green beans, trimmed and halved
- ½ cup beef stock
- 1 teaspoon sweet paprika
- ½ teaspoon chili powder
- A pinch of salt and black pepper
- 1 tablespoon lime juice
- 2 tablespoons parsley, chopped

Directions:
1. Heat up a pan with the oil over medium high heat, add the pork and brown for 5 minutes.
2. Add the stock and the other ingredients, toss, bring to a simmer and cook over medium heat for 25 minutes more.
3. Divide everything between plates and serve.

Nutrition:
calories 404, fat 34.5, fiber 2.6, carbs 5.2, protein 20

Chili Peppers Lamb Chops

Prep time: 10 minutes | **Cooking time:** 30 minutes | **Servings:** 2

Ingredients:
- 2 lamb chops
- 2 tablespoons ghee, melted
- Juice of 1 lime
- Zest of 1 lime, grated
- A pinch of salt and black pepper
- 2 chili peppers, chopped
- ½ cup beef stock
- ½ tablespoon chives, chopped

Directions:
1. Heat up a pan with the ghee over medium heat, add the lamb chops and brown for 5 minutes.
2. Add the rest of the ingredients, toss, introduce in the oven and cook at 390 degrees F for 25 minutes.
3. Divide the lamb chops mix between plates and serve.

Nutrition:
calories 450, fat 34, fiber 2, carbs 6, protein 26

Dill and Cayenne Pepper Beef

Prep time: 10 minutes | **Cooking time:** 30 minutes | **Servings:** 2

Ingredients:

- 1 pound beef stew meat, cubed
- 2 tablespoons ghee, melted
- A pinch of salt and black pepper
- 1 avocado, peeled, pitted and cubed
- 1 teaspoon sweet paprika
- ½ teaspoon coriander, ground
- 1 tablespoon dill, chopped
- A pinch of salt and black pepper
- A pinch of cayenne pepper
- ½ teaspoon garlic powder
- ½ cup beef stock

Directions:

1. Heat up a pan with the ghee over medium heat, add the meat and brown for 5 minutes.
2. Add the avocado and the rest of the ingredients, toss, cook for 25 minutes more, divide everything between plates and serve.

Nutrition:

calories 180, fat 5, fiber 1, carbs 5, protein 25

Meat Salad with Capers

Prep time: 10 minutes | **Cooking time:** 30 minutes | **Servings:** 2

Ingredients:

- 1 pound lamb shoulder, cut into strips
- 1 tablespoon olive oil
- 1 cup baby spinach
- 1 cup cherry tomatoes, halved
- 1 tablespoon capers, drained
- ¼ cup black olives, pitted and halved
- 2 scallions, chopped
- 1 tablespoon balsamic vinegar
- A pinch of salt and black pepper

Directions:

1. Heat up a pan with the oil over medium heat, add the scallions and the meat and brown for 5 minutes.
2. Add the rest of the ingredients except the spinach, toss and cook for 20 minutes more.
3. Add the spinach, toss, cook for 5 minutes, divide into bowls and serve.

Nutrition:

calories 250, fat 12, fiber 3, carbs 8, protein 18

Vinegar Beef

Prep time: 10 minutes | **Cooking time:** 30 minutes | **Servings:** 2

Ingredients:

- 2 tablespoons ghee
- 1 pound beef stew meat, cubed
- 1 cup spring onions, chopped
- 2 zucchinis, cubed
- 1 tablespoon balsamic vinegar
- 1 teaspoon sweet paprika
- 1 garlic clove, minced
- A pinch of salt and black pepper
- ½ cup beef stock

Directions:

1. Heat up a pan with the ghee over medium heat, add the spring onions and cook for 5 minutes.
2. Add the meat and cook for 5 minutes more.
3. Add the rest of the ingredients, toss, bring to a simmer and cook for 20 minutes.
4. Divide everything into bowls and serve.

Nutrition:

calories 204, fat 12, fiber 1, carbs 5, protein 10

Parsley Lamb Cubes

Prep time: 10 minutes | **Cooking time:** 30 minutes | **Servings:** 2

Ingredients:

- 1 pound lamb stew meat, cubed
- 2 tablespoons ghee, melted
- ½ teaspoon turmeric powder
- 1 tablespoon balsamic vinegar
- 2 garlic cloves, minced
- 2 teaspoons oregano, dried
- ½ teaspoon cumin, ground
- 2 tablespoons parsley, chopped
- A pinch of salt and black pepper

Directions:

1. Heat up a pan with the ghee over medium heat, add the garlic and the meat and brown for 5 minutes.
2. Add the vinegar and the other ingredients, toss, cook for 25 minutes more, divide between plates and serve with a side salad.

Nutrition:

calories 245, fat 32, fiber 6, carbs 4, protein 34

Mint Lamb Cubes

Prep time: 10 minutes | **Cooking time:** 30 minutes | **Servings:** 2

Ingredients:

- 1 tablespoon olive oil
- 1 pound lamb stew meat, cubed
- 1 tablespoon mint, chopped
- 3 scallions, chopped
- 2 garlic cloves, minced
- A pinch of salt and black pepper
- 2/3 cup heavy cream
- ½ teaspoon garam masala
- 1 tablespoon mustard

Directions:

1. Heat up a pan with the oil over medium heat, add the scallions and garlic and cook for 5 minutes.
2. Add the meat and brown for 5 minutes more.
3. Add the rest of the ingredients, toss, cook for 20 minutes more, divide into bowls and serve.

Nutrition:

calories 435, fat 30, fiber 4, carbs 5, protein 32

Garlic Cubed Pork

Prep time: 10 minutes | **Cooking time:** 35 minutes | **Servings:** 2

Ingredients:

- 1 pound pork stew meat, cubed
- 1 cup beef stock
- 1 cup cherry tomatoes, halved
- 1 tablespoon olive oil
- A pinch of salt and black pepper
- 1 teaspoon rosemary, dried
- 1 teaspoon sweet paprika
- 3 garlic cloves, minced
- A pinch of salt and black pepper
- 1 tablespoon chives, chopped

Directions:

1. Heat up a pan with the oil over medium heat, add the garlic and the meat and brown for 5 minutes.
2. Add the rest of the ingredients, toss, cook everything for 30 minutes more, divide between plates and serve.

Nutrition:

calories 578, fat 29.6, fiber 1.2, carbs 6.2, protein 69.1

Scallions Lamb Chops

Prep time: 10 minutes | **Cooking time:** 25 minutes | **Servings:** 2

Ingredients:

- 2 lamb chops
- 1 tablespoon olive oil
- 3 scallions, chopped
- A pinch of salt and black pepper
- ½ teaspoon red pepper flakes, crushed
- 1 tablespoon balsamic vinegar
- 1 tablespoon rosemary, chopped

Directions:

1. Heat up a pan with the oil over medium heat, add the scallions and the pepper flakes and cook for 5 minutes.
2. Add the lamb chops and brown for 5 minutes more.
3. Add the rest of the ingredients, toss, cook for 15 minutes more, divide between plates and serve.

Nutrition:

calories 684, fat 31.3, fiber 1.4, carbs 3.1, protein 92.4

Ketogenic Vegetable Recipes

Scallions Broccoli

Prep time: 10 minutes | **Cooking time:** 25 minutes | **Servings:** 2

Ingredients:

- ½ pound broccoli florets
- 3 scallions, chopped
- 2 garlic cloves, minced
- 2 tablespoons ghee, melted
- 1 tablespoon dill, chopped
- ½ teaspoon turmeric powder
- 1 teaspoon chili powder
- A pinch of salt and black pepper

Directions:

1. Heat up a pan with the ghee over medium heat, add the scallions and the garlic and cook for 5 minutes.
2. Add the broccoli and the other ingredients, toss, cook for 20 minutes more, divide between plates and serve.

Nutrition:

calories 173, fat 13.5, fiber 4.3, carbs 12.2, protein 4.3

Cilantro Brussels Sprouts

Prep time: 10 minutes | **Cooking time:** 20 minutes | **Servings:** 2

Ingredients:

- ½ pound Brussels sprouts, trimmed and halved
- 2 tablespoons ghee, melted
- 3 scallions, chopped
- ½ cup veggie stock
- ½ teaspoon rosemary, dried
- ½ teaspoon sweet paprika
- ½ teaspoon nutmeg, ground
- 1 teaspoon cilantro, chopped
- A pinch of salt and black pepper

Directions:

1. Heat up a pan with the ghee over medium heat, add the scallions, nutmeg and paprika, stir and cook for 5 minutes.
2. Add the sprouts and the other ingredients, toss, cook over medium heat for 15 minutes more, divide between plates and serve.

Nutrition:

calories 192, fat 18.8, fiber 1.2, carbs 5.1, protein 3.2

Tender Beef Roast

Prep time: 5 minutes | **Cooking time:** 45 minutes | **Servings:** 2

Ingredients:

- 1 pound beef roast, sliced
- 1 tablespoon balsamic vinegar
- 1 tablespoon olive oil
- 1 cup cherry tomatoes, halved
- 1 cup beef stock
- 1 red bell pepper, roughly cubed
- ½ teaspoon chili powder
- ½ teaspoon rosemary, dried
- A pinch of salt and black pepper

Directions:

1. Grease a baking dish with the oil, add the roast and the other ingredients inside and toss.
2. Bake at 390 degrees F for 45 minutes, divide everything between plates and serve.

Nutrition:

calories 150, fat 4, fiber 1, carbs 2, protein 12

Italian Seasoning and Pesto Lamb

Prep time: 10 minutes | **Cooking time:** 40 minutes | **Servings:** 2

Ingredients:

- 1 tablespoon avocado oil
- 1 pound lamb stew meat, cubed
- 2 tablespoons basil pesto
- 2 scallions, chopped
- A pinch of salt and black pepper
- 1 green chili, minced
- 1 cup cherry tomatoes, halved
- ½ teaspoon sweet paprika
- 1 teaspoon garlic powder
- 1 teaspoon Italian seasoning

Directions:

1. Heat up a pan with the oil over medium heat, add the scallions and the chili and cook for 5 minutes.
2. Add the meat and brown for 5 minutes more.
3. Add the rest of the ingredients, toss, cook everything for 30 minutes more, divide into bowls and serve.

Nutrition:

calories 524, fat 43, fiber 2, carbs 4, protein 26

Radish and Lamb Stew

Prep time: 10 minutes | **Cooking time:** 30 minutes | **Servings:** 2

Ingredients:

- 1 pound lamb stew meat, cubed
- 1 cup coconut cream
- 2 scallions, chopped
- 1 cup radishes, halved
- 2 tablespoons ghee, melted
- ½ teaspoon turmeric powder
- ¼ cup beef stock
- 1 tablespoon chives, chopped
- A pinch of salt and black pepper
- ½ teaspoon rosemary, dried

Directions:

1. Heat up a pan with the ghee over medium heat, add the scallions and the meat and cook for 5 minutes.
2. Add the rest of the ingredients, toss, cook everything for 25 more minutes, divide into bowls and serve.

Nutrition:

calories 291, fat 22, fiber 2, carbs 4, protein 17

Chili Powder Pork Stew Meat

Prep time: 10 minutes | **Cooking time:** 30 minutes | **Servings:** 2

Ingredients:

- 1 pound pork stew meat, cubed
- 2 tablespoons ghee, melted
- 1 tablespoon oregano, chopped
- 3 garlic cloves, minced
- A pinch of salt and black pepper
- ½ teaspoon chili powder

Directions:

1. Heat up a pan with the ghee over medium heat, add the garlic and the meat and brown for 5 minutes.
2. Add the rest of the ingredients, toss, cook for 25 minutes more, divide between plates and serve.

Nutrition:

calories 609, fat 35, fiber 1.3, carbs 3.3, protein 67.1

Parmesan and Scallions Lamb Chops

Prep time: 10 minutes | **Cooking time:** 40 minutes | **Servings:** 2

Ingredients:

- 2 lamb chops
- 2 tablespoons ghee
- 3 scallions, chopped
- ½ cup parmesan, grated
- A pinch of salt and black pepper
- ½ teaspoon paprika
- ¾ teaspoon cumin powder
- ¼ cup beef stock

Directions:

1. Grease a roasting pan with the ghee and combine the lamb with the other ingredients except the cheese inside.
2. Introduce in the oven, bake at 390 degrees F for 30 minutes, sprinkle the cheese, cook for 10 minutes more, divide between plates and serve.

Nutrition:

calories 200, fat 5, fiber 2, carbs 4, protein 8

Lamb with Capers

Prep time: 10 minutes | **Cooking time:** 40 minutes | **Servings:** 2

Ingredients:

- 1 pound lamb stew meat, cubed
- 1 tablespoon olive oil
- 1 tablespoon capers, drained
- 2 garlic cloves, minced
- 2 scallions, chopped
- A pinch of salt and black pepper
- ½ cup beef stock
- 1 teaspoon turmeric powder
- ½ teaspoon chili powder
- 1 tablespoon chives, chopped

Directions:

1. Heat up a pan with the oil over medium heat, add the scallions and garlic and cook for 5 minutes.
2. Add the meat and cook for another 5 minutes.
3. Add the rest of the ingredients, toss, cook for 30 minutes more, divide into bowls and serve.

Nutrition:

calories 276, fat 6, fiber 4, carbs 5, protein 36

Walnuts Salad

Prep time: 10 minutes | **Servings:** 2

Ingredients:

- ½ pound radishes, halved
- 1 cup baby spinach
- 1 cup cherry tomatoes, halved
- 1 tablespoon olive oil
- Juice of 1 lime
- 2 tablespoons walnuts, chopped
- 1 tablespoon balsamic vinegar
- Salt and black pepper to the taste

Directions:

1. 1. In a bowl, combine the radishes with the spinach, tomatoes and the other ingredients, toss and serve.

Nutrition:

calories 120, fat 2, fiber 1, carbs 4, protein 8

Tender Keto Salad

Prep time: 10 minutes | **Servings:** 2

Ingredients:

- 2 avocados, peeled, pitted and cubed
- 1 red bell pepper, roughly cubed
- 1 green bell pepper, roughly cubed
- 1 tablespoon olive oil
- 2 spring onions, chopped
- 1 tablespoon capers, drained
- 1 cup baby arugula
- 1 tablespoon chives, chopped
- A pinch of salt and black pepper

Directions:

1. In a bowl, combine the avocados with the peppers and the other ingredients, toss and serve.

Nutrition:

calories 234, fat 12, fiber 4, carbs 7, protein 12

Turmeric Sliced Zucchini Mix

Prep time: 10 minutes | **Cooking time:** 15 minutes | **Servings:** 2

Ingredients:

- 2 zucchinis, sliced
- Juice of 1 lemon
- 2 tablespoons avocado oil
- A pinch of salt and black pepper
- ½ teaspoon turmeric powder
- 1 garlic clove, minced
- 1 tablespoon chives, chopped

Directions:

1. Heat up a pan with the oil over medium heat, add the garlic and cook for 2 minutes.
2. Add the zucchinis and the other ingredients, toss, cook for 13 minutes more, divide between plates and serve.

Nutrition:

calories 154, fat 12, fiber 3, carbs 5, protein 4

Pork with Sliced Fennel

Prep time: 10 minutes | **Cooking time:** 30 minutes | **Servings:** 2

Ingredients:

- 1 pound pork stew meat, cubed
- 2 tablespoons ghee, melted
- 1 fennel bulb, sliced
- A pinch of salt and black pepper
- ½ teaspoon cumin, ground
- ½ teaspoon sweet paprika
- 1 teaspoon oregano, dried
- ½ cup beef stock

Directions:

1. Heat up a pan with the ghee over medium heat, add the meat and brown for 5 minutes.
2. Add the fennel and the other ingredients, toss, cook for 25 minutes more, divide between plates and serve.

Nutrition:

calories 264, fat 14, fiber 3, carbs 5, protein 24

Garlic Peppers

Prep time: 10 minutes | **Cooking time:** 20 minutes | **Servings:** 2

Ingredients:

- 1 red bell pepper, cut into strips
- 1 green bell pepper, cut into strips
- 1 orange bell pepper, cut into strips
- 1 cup heavy cream
- 4 scallions, chopped
- 2 tablespoons olive oil
- 2 garlic cloves, minced
- A pinch of salt and black pepper
- 1 teaspoon turmeric powder
- 1 tablespoon chives, chopped

Directions:

1. Heat up a pan with the oil over medium heat, add the scallions and the garlic and cook for 5 minutes.
2. Add the bell peppers and cook for 5 minutes more.
3. Add the rest of the ingredients, toss, cook for 10 minutes more, divide everything between plates and serve.

Nutrition:

calories 176, fat 13, fiber 1, carbs 4, protein 6

Garam Masala Green Cabbage

Prep time: 10 minutes | **Cooking time:** 25 minutes | **Servings:** 2

Ingredients:

- ½ pound green cabbage, shredded
- 2 tablespoons ghee
- 1 teaspoon cumin, ground
- 3 scallions, chopped
- ½ teaspoon sweet paprika
- ½ teaspoon garam masala
- ¼ cup veggie stock
- 1 tablespoon dill, chopped

Directions:

1. Heat up a pan with the ghee over medium heat, add the scallions and the cumin and cook for 5 minutes.
2. Add the cabbage and cook for 5 minutes more.
3. Add the rest of the ingredients, toss, cook for 15 minutes, divide into bowls and serve.

Nutrition:

calories 200, fat 3, fiber 2, carbs 6, protein 8

Broccoli Spread

Prep time: 10 minutes | **Cooking time:** 20 minutes | **Servings:** 2

Ingredients:

- ½ pound broccoli florets
- 2 cups veggie stock
- 1 tablespoon avocado oil
- 1 teaspoon chili powder
- 3 scallions, chopped
- A pinch of salt and black pepper
- A pinch of red pepper flakes, crushed
- 2 garlic cloves, minced

Directions:

1. Heat up a pot with the oil over medium heat, add the scallions and the garlic and cook for 3 minutes.
2. Add the broccoli and cook for 2-3 minutes more.
3. Add the rest of the ingredients, toss, cook for 15 minutes, blend using an immersion blender, divide into bowls and serve.

Nutrition:

calories 230, fat 3, fiber 3, carbs 6, protein 10

Cumin Swiss Chard with Kalamata Olives

Prep time: 10 minutes | **Cooking time:** 25 minutes | **Servings:** 2

Ingredients:

- 2 cups Swiss chard, chopped
- 3 scallions, chopped
- ½ cup kalamata olives, pitted and halved
- 1 tablespoon olive oil
- 4 garlic cloves, minced
- A pinch of salt and black pepper
- ½ teaspoon sweet paprika
- ½ teaspoon cumin, ground

Directions:

1. Heat up a pan with the oil over medium heat, add the scallions and the garlic and cook for 5 minutes.
2. Add the Swiss chard and the other ingredients, toss, cook for 20 minutes more, divide between plates and serve.

Nutrition:

calories 332, fat 23, fiber 3, carbs 4, protein 23

Tender Cilantro Lamb Chops

Prep time: 10 minutes | **Cooking time:** 35 minutes | **Servings:** 2

Ingredients:

- 1 pound lamb chops
- 2 tablespoons ghee
- 1 teaspoon coriander, ground
- ½ teaspoon sweet paprika
- ½ cup beef stock
- A pinch of salt and black pepper
- 2 garlic cloves, minced
- 2 tablespoons cilantro, chopped

Directions:

1. Heat up a pan with the ghee over medium heat, add the garlic and the lamb chops and brown for 5 minutes.
2. Add the rest of the ingredients, toss, introduce in the oven and cook at 390 degrees F for 30 minutes.
3. Divide everything between plates and serve.

Nutrition:

calories 250, fat 5, fiber 1, carbs 5, protein 8

Garam Masala Brussels Sprouts

Prep time: 10 minutes | **Cooking time:** 20 minutes | **Servings:** 2

Ingredients:

- 2 cups Brussels sprouts, trimmed and halved
- 3 scallions, chopped
- 1 tablespoon ginger, grated
- ¼ cup vegetable stock
- 1 tablespoon olive oil
- ½ teaspoon rosemary, dried
- ½ teaspoon garam masala
- A pinch of salt and black pepper

Directions:

1. Heat up a pan with the oil over medium heat, add the scallions and the ginger and cook for 5 minutes.
2. Add the sprouts and the other ingredients, toss, cook for 15 minutes more, divide between plates and serve.

Nutrition:

calories 140, fat 2, fiber 1, carbs 3, protein 7

Garam Masala Beef with Artichokes

Prep time: 10 minutes | **Cooking time:** 30 minutes | **Servings:** 2

Ingredients:

- 1 pound beef stew meat, cubed
- 1 tablespoon ghee, melted
- 1 teaspoon sweet paprika
- 2 small artichokes, trimmed and quartered
- ½ cup beef stock
- A pinch of salt and black pepper
- 2 tablespoons chives, chopped
- ½ teaspoon garam masala
- ¼ teaspoon garlic powder

Directions:

1. Heat up a pan with the ghee over medium heat, add the meat and brown for 5 minutes.
2. Add the paprika, artichokes and the other ingredients, toss, cook for 25 minutes more, divide between plates and serve.

Nutrition:

calories 275, fat 7, fiber 2, carbs 4, protein 10

Cumin and Chili Powder Lamb Chops

Prep time: 10 minutes | **Cooking time:** 30 minutes | **Servings:** 2

Ingredients:

- 1 tablespoon olive oil
- 2 lamb chops
- 1 cup cherry tomatoes, halved
- 3 garlic cloves, minced
- A pinch of salt and black pepper
- ½ cup beef stock
- ½ teaspoon chili powder
- 1 teaspoon cumin, ground
- 1 tablespoon chives, chopped

Directions:

1. Grease a baking pan with the oil and add the lamb chops inside.
2. Add the rest of the ingredients, toss and bake at 390 degrees F for 30 minutes.
3. Divide everything between plates and serve.

Nutrition:

calories 334, fat 33, fiber 3, carbs 5, protein 7

Kale and Ground Beef

Prep time: 10 minutes | **Cooking time:** 25 minutes | **Servings:** 2

Ingredients:

- 1 pound beef meat, ground
- ½ cup kalamata olives, pitted and halved
- 1 cup baby kale
- 1 tablespoon olive oil
- ½ teaspoon chili powder
- ½ teaspoon sweet paprika
- ½ cup beef stock
- 2 garlic cloves, minced
- A pinch of salt and black pepper

Directions:

1. Heat up a pan with the oil over medium heat, add the garlic and the meat and brown for 5 minutes.
2. Add the rest of the ingredients, toss, cook for 20 minutes more, divide into bowls and serve.

Nutrition:

calories 435, fat 23, fiber 4, carbs 6, protein 32

Turmeric Bok Choy

Prep time: 10 minutes | **Cooking time:** 20 minutes | **Servings:** 2

Ingredients:

- ½ pound bok choy
- 3 scallions, chopped
- 1 tablespoon olive oil
- 1 teaspoon rosemary, dried
- ½ teaspoon turmeric powder
- 1 tablespoon balsamic vinegar
- ½ cup vegetable stock
- A pinch of salt and black pepper

Directions:

1. Heat up a pan with the oil over medium heat, add the scallions and the turmeric and cook for 5 minutes.
2. Add the bok choy and the other ingredients, toss, cook for 15 minutes more, divide between plates and serve.

Nutrition:

calories 120, fat 8, fiber 1, carbs 3, protein 7

Garam Masala Lamb

Prep time: 10 minutes | **Cooking time:** 30 minutes | **Servings:** 2

Ingredients:

- 1 pound lamb stew meat, cubed
- 1 tablespoon olive oil
- 1 teaspoon chili powder
- A pinch of salt and black pepper
- ½ teaspoon garam masala
- ½ teaspoon coriander, ground
- 1 cup beef stock
- ¼ cup tomato passata (unsweetened)

Directions:

1. Heat up a pan with the oil over medium heat, add the meat and brown for 5 minutes.
2. Add the rest of the ingredients, toss, cook for 25 minutes more, divide between plates and serve.

Nutrition:

calories 494, fat 24.1, fiber 0.5, carbs 0.8, protein 65.2

Coconut Cream Beef

Prep time: 10 minutes | **Cooking time:** 30 minutes | **Servings:** 2

Ingredients:

- 1 pound beef stew meat, cubed
- 1 tablespoon olive oil
- 3 scallions, chopped
- 1 cup coconut cream
- A pinch of salt and black pepper
- 2 garlic cloves, minced
- 1 tablespoon chili powder

Directions:

1. Heat up a pan with the oil over medium heat, add the scallions and the garlic and cook for 5 minutes.
2. Add the meat and cook for 5 minutes more.
3. Add the rest of the ingredients, toss and cook for 20 minutes more.
4. Divide everything between plates and serve.

Nutrition:

calories 200, fat 8, fiber 1, carbs 5.3, protein 26

Ginger and Rosemary Broccoli

Prep time: 10 minutes | **Cooking time:** 30 minutes | **Servings:** 2

Ingredients:

- ½ pound broccoli florets
- 1 tablespoon olive oil
- 2 spring onions, chopped
- 1 tablespoon ginger, grated
- 1 tablespoon lime juice
- ½ teaspoon rosemary, dried
- ½ teaspoon chili powder
- ¼ cup veggie stock
- 2 garlic cloves, minced

Directions:

1. Heat up a pan with the oil over medium heat, add the spring onions, ginger and garlic and cook for 5 minutes.
2. Add the broccoli and the other ingredients, toss, cook for 25 minutes more, divide between plates and serve.

Nutrition:

calories 150, fat 4, fiber 2, carbs 5, protein 12

Passata Pork Chops

Prep time: 10 minutes | **Cooking time:** 25 minutes | **Servings:** 2

Ingredients:

- 2 pork chops
- 1 tablespoon olive oil
- 1 cup cherry tomatoes, halved
- 1 cup tomato passata (unsweetened)
- A pinch of salt and black pepper
- 1 tablespoon rosemary, chopped
- 1 teaspoon cumin, ground

Directions:

1. Heat up a pan with the oil over medium high heat, add the pork chops and brown for 5 minutes.
2. Add the rest of the ingredients, toss and cook for 20 minutes more.
3. Divide the mix between plates and serve.

Nutrition:

calories 210, fat 10, fiber 2, carbs 6, protein 19

Tender Sour Lamb Riblets

Prep time: 10 minutes | **Cooking time:** 1 hour

Servings: 2

Ingredients:

- ½ cup parsley
- 3 scallions, chopped
- 2 tablespoons walnuts, chopped
- 1 teaspoon lemon zest, grated
- 1 teaspoon lemon juice
- 2 tablespoons avocado oil
- 1 pound lamb riblets
- A pinch of salt and black pepper

Directions:

1. In your food processor, combine the parsley with the scallions and the other ingredients except the lamb and the stock and pulse well.
2. In a roasting pan, combine the lamb with the parsley mix and the stock, toss and cook at 390 degrees F for 1 hour.
3. Divide between plates and serve.

Nutrition:

calories 200, fat 4, fiber 1, carbs 5, protein 7

Tomato Passata Kale

Prep time: 10 minutes | **Cooking time:** 20 minutes | **Servings:** 2

Ingredients:

- 3 scallions, chopped
- 1 pound kale, roughly torn
- 2 tablespoons ghee, melted
- 1 teaspoon sweet paprika
- ½ cup tomato passata (unsweetened)
- A pinch of salt and black pepper
- 3 garlic cloves, minced
- ½ tablespoon red pepper flakes, crushed
- 1 tablespoon chives, chopped

Directions:

1. Heat up a pan with the ghee over medium heat, add the scallions and the garlic and cook for 5 minutes.
2. Add the kale and the other ingredients, toss, cook for 15 minutes more, divide between plates and serve.

Nutrition:

calories 246, fat 13.2, fiber 4.9, carbs 28.3, protein 7.9

Rosemary Lamb

Prep time: 10 minutes | **Cooking time:** 30 minutes | **Servings:** 2

Ingredients:

- 1 pound lamb stew meat, cubed
- 1 teaspoon turmeric powder
- 1 tablespoon ghee, melted
- 3 scallions, chopped
- A pinch of salt and black pepper
- 1 tablespoon chives, chopped
- 1 cup beef stock
- ½ teaspoon rosemary, dried

Directions:

1. Heat up a pan with the ghee over medium heat, add the scallions and the meat and brown for 5 minutes.
2. Add the rest of the ingredients, toss, cook for 25 minutes more, divide between plates and serve.

Nutrition:

calories 325, fat 18, fiber 1, carbs 5.6, protein 36

Cumin Cauliflower

Prep time: 10 minutes | **Cooking time:** 25 minutes | **Servings:** 2

Ingredients:

- 1 pound cauliflower florets
- 2 tablespoons ghee, melted
- 1 cup coconut cream
- 1 tablespoon chives, chopped
- 2 spring onions, chopped
- 2 garlic cloves, minced
- A pinch of salt and black pepper
- 1 cup vegetable stock
- ½ teaspoon cumin, ground

Directions:

1. Heat up a pan with the ghee over medium heat, add the onions and the garlic and cook for 5 minutes.
2. Add the cauliflower and the other ingredients, toss, cook everything fro 20 minutes more, divide between plates and serve.

Nutrition:

calories 457, fat 41.7, fiber 8.9, carbs 21.1, protein 7.9

Coconut Aminos Pork

Prep time: 10 minutes | **Cooking time:** 30 minutes | **Servings:** 2

Ingredients:

- 1 pound stew meat, cubed
- A pinch of salt and black pepper
- ½ teaspoon chili powder
- 1 tablespoon ghee, melted
- 1 cup coconut cream
- 2 tablespoons coconut aminos
- A pinch of salt and black pepper
- 1 tablespoon parsley, chopped

Directions:

1. Heat up a pan with the ghee over medium heat, add the meat and brown for 5 minutes.
2. Add the rest of the ingredients, toss, cook for 25 minutes more, divide into bowls and serve.

Nutrition:

calories 137, fat 6, fiber 2, carbs 5, protein 17

Cumin Pork Chops

Prep time: 10 minutes | **Cooking time:** 25 minutes | **Servings:** 2

Ingredients:

- 2 pork chops
- 1 cup shallot, chopped
- ¼ cup beef stock
- 2 tablespoons ghee, melted
- 1 teaspoon cumin, ground
- A pinch of salt and black pepper
- ½ teaspoon rosemary, dried

Directions:

1. Heat up a pan with the ghee over medium heat, add the shallots and cook for 5 minutes.
2. Add the pork chops and brown for 5 minutes more.
3. Add the rest of the ingredients, toss, cook for 15 minutes more, divide between plates and serve.

Nutrition:

calories 132, fat 5, fiber 1, carbs 1, protein 18

Rosemary Beef with Swiss Chard

Prep time: 10 minutes | **Cooking time:** 35 minutes | **Servings:** 2

Ingredients:

- 1 pound beef stew meat, cubed
- 1 tablespoon olive oil
- 1 cup Swiss chard, torn
- 2 scallions, chopped
- ½ teaspoon chili powder
- ½ teaspoon rosemary, dried
- ½ cup beef stock
- A pinch of salt and black pepper

Directions:

1. Heat up a pot with the oil over medium heat, add the scallions and cook for 2 minutes.
2. Add the meat and brown for 3 minutes more.
3. Add the rest of the ingredients, toss, cook for 30 minutes more, divide between plates and serve.

Nutrition:

calories 230, fat 7, fiber 4, carbs 6, protein 29

Chili Lamb with Mushrooms

Prep time: 10 minutes | **Cooking time:** 35 minutes | **Servings:** 2

Ingredients:

- 1 tablespoon olive oil
- 2 scallions, chopped
- 2 garlic cloves, minced
- 1 pound lamb chops
- 1 cup baby Bella mushrooms, halved
- ½ cup beef stock
- A pinch of salt and black pepper
- ½ teaspoon sweet paprika
- ½ teaspoon chili powder

Directions:

1. In a roasting pan, combine the lamb chops with the scallions, garlic and the other ingredients, toss and bake at 390 degrees F for 35 minutes.
2. Divide everything between plates and serve.

Nutrition:

calories 435, fat 16, fiber 1, carbs 7, protein 45

Rosemary Pork Cubes

Prep time: 10 minutes | **Cooking time:** 30 minutes | **Servings:** 2

Ingredients:

- 1 pound pork stew meat, cubed
- 1 tablespoon olive oil
- 3 garlic cloves, minced
- 1 tablespoon rosemary, chopped
- 1 cup beef stock
- 1 teaspoon sweet paprika
- A pinch of salt and black pepper

Directions:

1. Heat up a pan with the oil over medium heat, add the garlic and the meat and brown for 5 minutes.
2. Add the rest of the ingredients, toss, cook for 25 minutes more, divide between plates and serve.

Nutrition:

calories 165, fat 2, fiber 1, carbs 2, protein 26

Cumin Pork with Avocado

Prep time: 10 minutes | **Cooking time:** 30 minutes | **Servings:** 2

Ingredients:

- 1 pound pork stew meat, cubed
- 1 tablespoon avocado oil
- 1 avocado, peeled, pitted and cubed
- 1 teaspoon chili powder
- A pinch of salt and black pepper
- ½ teaspoon cumin, ground
- ½ cup beef stock

Directions:

1. Heat up a pan with the oil over medium heat, add the meat and chili powder and brown for 5 minutes.
2. Add the rest of the ingredients, toss, cook for 25 minutes more, divide between plates and serve,

Nutrition:

calories 643, fat 37.1, fiber 1.5, carbs 3.3, protein 71.8

Chili Beef with Tarragon

Prep time: 10 minutes | **Cooking time:** 30 minutes | **Servings:** 2

Ingredients:

- 1 pound beef stew meat, cubed
- 1 tablespoon ghee, melted
- 1 tablespoon tarragon, chopped
- A pinch of salt and black pepper
- 1 teaspoon cumin, ground
- 1 teaspoon chili powder
- ¼ cup beef stock

Directions:

1. Heat up a pan with the ghee over medium heat, add the meat and brown for 5 minutes.
2. Add the rest of the ingredients, toss, cook for 25 minutes more, divide between plates and serve.

Nutrition:

calories 700, fat 56, fiber 2, carbs 13.10, protein 70

Dill Mix

Prep time: 10 minutes | **Cooking time:** 15 minutes | **Servings:** 2

Ingredients:

- 2 zucchinis, roughly cubed
- 1 cup black olives, pitted and halved
- ½ cup kalamata olives, pitted and halved
- 1 tablespoon olive oil
- ½ teaspoon chili powder
- ½ teaspoon sweet paprika
- 1 tablespoon dill, chopped
- A pinch of salt and black pepper
- 1 tablespoon balsamic vinegar

Directions:

1. Heat up a pan with the oil over medium heat, add the olives and the zucchinis and cook for 5 minutes.
2. Add the rest of the ingredients, toss gently, cook for 10 minutes more, divide between plates and serve.

Nutrition:

calories 200, fat 13, fiber 3, carbs 5, protein 7

Aromatic Lamb Chops

Prep time: 10 minutes | **Cooking time:** 30 minutes | **Servings:** 2

Ingredients:

- 1 pound lamb chops
- 2 tablespoons ghee, melted
- A pinch of salt and black pepper
- 1 teaspoon chili powder
- ½ cup beef stock
- 1 tablespoon mint, chopped

Directions:

1. Heat up a pan with the ghee over medium heat, add the meat and brown for 5 minutes.
2. Add the rest of the ingredients, toss, bring to a simmer and cook over medium heat for 25 minutes more.
3. Divide everything between plates and serve.

Nutrition:

calories 200, fat 4, fiber 1, carbs 3, protein 7

Tender Beef Stew Meat

Prep time: 10 minutes | **Cooking time:** 25 minutes | **Servings:** 2

Ingredients:

- 1 pound beef stew meat, cubed
- 1 cup red bell peppers, cubed
- 1 tablespoon olive oil
- 1 tablespoon rosemary, chopped
- ½ teaspoon cumin, ground
- A pinch of salt and black pepper
- 1 teaspoon sweet paprika

Directions:

1. Heat up a pan with the oil over medium heat, add the meat and brown for 5 minutes.
2. Add the peppers and the other ingredients, toss, cook for 20 minutes more, divide between plates and serve.

Nutrition:

calories 250, fat 5, fiber 1, carbs 3, protein 12

Fennel Mix

Prep time: 10 minutes | **Cooking time:** 20 minutes | **Servings:** 2

Ingredients:

- 2 fennel bulbs, sliced
- 1 cup Brussels sprouts, trimmed and halved
- 1 tablespoon olive oil
- 1 tablespoon lime juice
- 1 tablespoon onion flakes
- A pinch of salt and black pepper
- ½ teaspoon chili powder
- 1 tablespoon chives, chopped

Directions:

1. Spread the fennel and the Brussels sprouts on a baking sheet lined with parchment paper, add the rest of the ingredients, toss and bake at 390 degrees F for 20 minutes.
2. Divide everything between plates and serve.

Nutrition:

calories 140, fat 2, fiber 1, carbs 5, protein 10

Creamy Sprouts

Prep time: 10 minutes | **Cooking time:** 25 minutes | **Servings:** 2

Ingredients:

- 1 cup bok choy, torn
- 1 cup Brussels sprouts, trimmed and halved
- 2 tablespoons ghee, melted
- A pinch of salt and black pepper
- 2 garlic cloves, minced
- A pinch of salt and black pepper
- ¾ cup heavy cream
- 1 tablespoon dill, chopped

Directions:

1. Heat up a pot with the ghee over medium high heat, add the garlic and cook for 2 minutes.
2. Add the sprouts, bok choy and the other ingredients, toss, cook over medium heat for 23 minutes more, divide between plates and serve.

Nutrition:

calories 150, fat 3, fiber 1, carbs 2, protein 6

Lemon and Coriander Brussels Sprouts

Prep time: 10 minutes | **Cooking time:** 25 minutes | **Servings:** 2

Ingredients:

- ½ pound Brussels sprouts, trimmed and halved
- 1 bunch green onion, chopped
- 2 garlic cloves, minced
- A pinch of salt and black pepper
- ½ teaspoon cumin, ground
- ½ teaspoon coriander, ground
- Juice of ½ lemon
- Zest of ½ lemon, grated
- 1 tablespoon olive oil

Directions:

3. In a roasting pan, combine the sprouts with the green onions, garlic and the other ingredients, toss and bake at 390 degrees F for 25 minutes.
4. Divide everything between plates and serve.

Nutrition:

calories 170, fat 7, fiber 4, carbs 6, protein 10

Red Chili Baby Spinach

Prep time: 10 minutes | **Cooking time:** 12 minutes | **Servings:** 2

Ingredients:

- 2 tablespoons ghee
- 1 pound baby spinach
- 1 red chili, minced
- ½ teaspoon chili powder
- 2 garlic cloves, minced
- ¼ cup veggie stock
- A pinch of salt and black pepper
- 1 tablespoon cilantro, chopped

Directions:

1. Heat up a pan with the ghee over medium heat, add the garlic and chili and cook for 2 minutes.
2. Add the spinach and the other ingredients, toss, cook for 10 minutes more, divide between plates and serve.

Nutrition:

calories 245, fat 24, fiber 3, carbs 4, protein 6

Rosemary Green Beans

Prep time: 10 minutes | **Cooking time:** 20 minutes | **Servings:** 2

Ingredients:

- 1 pound green beans, trimmed and halved
- 1 tablespoon olive oil
- 3 garlic cloves, minced
- 1 tablespoon dill, chopped
- 1 cup veggie stock
- A pinch of salt and black pepper
- ½ teaspoon rosemary, dried
- ½ teaspoon cumin, ground
- 1 tablespoon cilantro, chopped

Directions:

1. Heat up a pan with the oil over medium heat, add the garlic and cumin and cook for 2 minutes.
2. Add the green beans and the other ingredients, toss, cook for 18 minutes more, divide between plates and serve.

Nutrition:

calories 144, fat 7.5, fiber 8.2, carbs 19, protein 4.9

Sesame and Coriander Kale

Prep time: 10 minutes | **Cooking time:** 20 minutes | **Servings:** 2

Ingredients:

- 1 pound baby kale
- 2 tablespoons ghee, melted
- 3 scallions, chopped
- ½ teaspoon coriander, ground
- ½ teaspoon chili powder
- ¼ cup veggie stock
- 1 teaspoon sesame seeds
- A pinch of salt and black pepper

Directions:

1. Heat up a pan with the ghee over medium heat, add the scallions and chili powder and cook for 5 minutes.
2. Add the kale and the other ingredients, toss, cook for 15 minutes more, divide into bowls and serve.

Nutrition:

calories 50, fat 1, fiber 0, carbs 1, protein 5

Cubed Avocado and Pork

Prep time: 10 minutes | **Cooking time:** 35 minutes | **Servings:** 2

Ingredients:

- 1 pound pork stew meat, cubed
- 1 tablespoon avocado oil
- 2 avocados, peeled, pitted and cubed
- 1 tablespoon capers, drained
- ½ cup beef stock
- ½ teaspoon sweet paprika
- ½ teaspoon rosemary, dried
- A pinch of salt and black pepper

Directions:

1. Heat up a pan with the oil over medium heat, add the meat and brown for 5 minutes.
2. Add the rest of the ingredients, toss, cook for 30 minutes more, divide the mix between plates and serve.

Nutrition:

calories 130, fat 12, fiber 1, carbs 3, protein 9

Cilantro Swiss Chard

Prep time: 10 minutes | **Cooking time:** 20 minutes | **Servings:** 2

Ingredients:

- 1 pound Swiss chard, torn
- 2 tablespoons ghee, melted
- 2 garlic cloves, minced
- A pinch of salt and black pepper
- 2 teaspoons balsamic vinegar
- ½ teaspoon chili powder
- 1 tablespoon cilantro, chopped

Directions:

1. Heat up a pan with the ghee over medium heat, add the garlic and cook for 2 minutes.
2. Add the Swiss chard and the other ingredients, toss, cook for 18 minutes more, divide between plates and serve.

Nutrition:

calories 164, fat 13.5, fiber 4.1, carbs 9.9, protein 4.4

Nutmeg Cauliflower

Prep time: 10 minutes | **Cooking time:** 20 minutes | **Servings:** 2

Ingredients:

- 2 garlic cloves, minced
- 1 tablespoon olive oil
- 2 cup cauliflower florets
- 1 tablespoon rosemary, dried
- ½ cup veggie stock
- ½ teaspoon hot paprika
- ½ teaspoon nutmeg, ground
- A pinch of salt and black pepper

Directions:

1. Heat up a pan with the oil over medium heat, add the garlic and cook for 2 minutes.
2. Add the cauliflower and the other ingredients, toss, cook for 18 minutes more, divide between plates and serve.

Nutrition:

calories 98, fat 7.6, fiber 3.4, carbs 7.7, protein 2.3

Lime Juice Lamb Chops

Prep time: 10 minutes | **Cooking time:** 40 minutes | **Servings:** 2

Ingredients:

- 2 lamb chops
- 2 endives, trimmed and shredded
- 2 tablespoons ghee, melted
- 2 scallions, chopped
- 2 garlic cloves, minced
- A pinch of salt and black pepper
- 1 tablespoon lime juice

Directions:

1. In a roasting pan, combine the lamb chops with the endives and the other ingredients, toss and cook at 390 degrees F for 40 minutes.
2. Divide everything between plates and serve.

Nutrition:

calories 230, fat 3, fiber 3, carbs 5, protein 10

Succulent Beef

Prep time: 10 minutes | **Cooking time:** 30 minutes | **Servings:** 2

Ingredients:

- 1 pound beef stew meat cubed
- 2 garlic cloves, minced
- Juice of 1 lemon
- Zest of ½ lemon, grated
- 2 tablespoons olive oil
- A pinch of salt and black pepper
- A handful parsley, chopped

Directions:

1. Heat up a pan with the oil over medium high heat, add the meat and brown for 5 minutes.
2. Add the rest of the ingredients, cook for 25 minutes more, stirring from time to time, divide between plates and serve.

Nutrition:

calories 250, fat 6, fiber 1, carbs 7, protein 33

Rosemary Sprouts with Avocado

Prep time: 10 minutes | **Cooking time:** 20 minutes | **Servings:** 2

Ingredients:

- 2 avocados, peeled, pitted and cubed
- 1 cup Brussels sprouts, trimmed and halved
- 1 tablespoon olive oil
- 2 scallions, chopped
- 1 tablespoon lime juice
- A pinch of salt and black pepper
- ½ teaspoon rosemary, dried

Directions:

1. Heat up a pan with the oil over medium heat, add the scallions and cook for 5 minutes.
2. Add the avocados and the other ingredients, toss, cook for 15 minutes more, divide into bowls and serve.

Nutrition:

calories 100, fat 10, fiber 2, carbs 5, protein 8

Lemon Lamb

Prep time: 10 minutes | **Cooking time:** 30 minutes | **Servings:** 2

Ingredients:

- 2 lamb chops
- 1 tablespoon olive oil
- 1 tablespoon oregano, chopped
- A pinch of salt and black pepper
- Zest of ½ lemon, grated
- ¼ cup beef stock

Directions:

1. In a roasting pan, combine the lamb chops with the oil and the other ingredients, toss and bake at 390 degrees F for 30 minutes.
2. Divide between plates and serve with a side salad.

Nutrition:

calories 160, fat 7, fiber 3, carbs 5, protein 12

Garlic Okra

Prep time: 10 minutes | **Cooking time:** 20 minutes | **Servings:** 2

Ingredients:

- 2 garlic cloves, minced
- 2 shallots, chopped
- 1 tablespoon avocado oil
- 2 cups okra, sliced
- Juice of 1 lime
- Zest of 1 lime, grated
- A pinch of salt and black pepper
- 1 tablespoon chives, chopped

Directions:

1. Heat up a pan with the oil over medium heat, add the shallots and the garlic and cook for 2 minutes.
2. Add the okra and the other ingredients, toss, cook for 18 minutes more, divide between plate sand serve.

Nutrition:

calories 89, fat 3.8, fiber 5.1, carbs 13.5, protein 2.9

Baby Spinach Bowl

Prep time: 10 minutes | **Cooking time:** 15 minutes | **Servings:** 2

Ingredients:

- 2 cups baby spinach
- 1 tablespoon pine nuts, toasted
- 2 scallions, chopped
- 1 tablespoon olive oil
- ½ teaspoon sweet paprika
- ½ teaspoon coriander, ground
- ¼ cup tomato passata (unsweetened)
- 1 tablespoon cilantro, chopped

Directions:

1. Heat up a pan with the oil over medium heat, add the scallions and cook for 2 minutes.
2. Add the spinach and the other ingredients, toss, cook for 13 minutes more, divide between plates and serve.

Nutrition:

calories 120, fat 1, fiber 2, carbs 3, protein 6

Cabbage and Scallions

Prep time: 10 minutes | **Servings:** 2

Ingredients:

- 3 scallions, chopped
- 1 green cabbage head, shredded
- 1 avocado, peeled, pitted and cubed
- 1 tablespoon olive oil
- ½ cup cherry tomatoes, halved
- 1 tablespoon lime juice
- ½ tablespoon lime zest, grated
- 1 tablespoon chives, chopped
- A pinch of salt and black pepper

Directions:

1. In a bowl, combine the cabbage with the avocado and the other ingredients, toss and serve cold.

Nutrition:

calories 151, fat 6, fiber 3, carbs 7, protein 8

Keto Vegetables Stew

Prep time: 10 minutes | **Cooking time:** 20 minutes | **Servings:** 2

Ingredients:

- 2 leeks, sliced
- 1 cup okra, sliced
- 1 tablespoon olive oil
- 3 garlic cloves, minced
- ½ teaspoon chili powder
- ½ cup tomato passata (unsweetened)
- A pinch of salt and black pepper
- 1 tablespoon chives, chopped

Directions:

1. Heat up a pan with the oil over medium heat, add the garlic and cook fro 2 minutes.
2. Add the okra, leeks and the other ingredients, toss, cook for 18 minutes more, divide between plates and serve.

Nutrition:

calories 144, fat 7.5, fiber 3.6, carbs 18.3, protein 2.7

Oregano Endives

Prep time: 10 minutes | **Cooking time:** 20 minutes | **Servings:** 2

Ingredients:

- 2 endives, shredded
- 2 tablespoons ghee, melted
- 3 garlic cloves, minced
- ½ cup veggie stock
- A pinch of salt and black pepper
- ½ teaspoon oregano, dried
- ½ teaspoon garam masala
- 1 tablespoon dill, chopped

Directions:

1. Heat up a pan with the ghee over medium heat, add the garlic and cook for 2 minutes.
2. Add the endives and the other ingredients, toss, cook for 18 minutes more, divide between plates and serve.

Nutrition:

calories 124, fat 12.9, fiber 0.5, carbs 2.6, protein 0.7

Soft Ghee Lamb

Prep time: 10 minutes | **Cooking time:** 45 minutes | **Servings:** 2

Ingredients:

- 1 pound lamb stew meat, cubed
- 2 tablespoons ghee
- 3 garlic cloves, minced
- 1 teaspoon sage, dried
- ½ teaspoon garam masala
- ½ teaspoon turmeric powder
- ½ cup beef stock
- A pinch of salt and black pepper
- 1 teaspoon Italian seasoning

Directions:

1. Heat up a pan with the ghee over medium heat, add the garlic and the meat and cook for 5 minutes.
2. Add the rest of the ingredients, toss, cook everything for 40 minutes more, divide into bowls and serve.

Nutrition:

calories 362, fat 21, fiber 2, carbs 6, protein 26

Garlic and Scallions Bok Choy

Prep time: 10 minutes | **Cooking time:** 12 minutes | **Servings:** 2

Ingredients:

- 2 cups bok choy
- 1 tablespoon avocado oil
- 1 teaspoon sage, dried
- Juice of 1 lime
- ½ teaspoon sweet paprika
- A pinch of salt and black pepper
- 2 scallions, chopped
- 1 garlic clove, minced

Directions:

1. Heat up a pan with the oil over medium heat, add the scallions and the garlic and cook for 2 minutes.
2. Add the bok choy and the other ingredients, toss, cook for 10 minutes more, divide between plates and serve.

Nutrition:

calories 120, fat 2, fiber 1, carbs 4, protein 5

Chard Bowl

Prep time: 10 minutes | **Cooking time:** 20 minutes | **Servings:** 2

Ingredients:

- 2 cups Swiss chard, chopped
- 1 zucchini, cubed
- 1 tablespoon olive oil
- 1 cup cherry tomatoes, halved
- 1 tablespoon balsamic vinegar
- 1 tablespoon chives, chopped
- A pinch of salt and black pepper

Directions:

1. Heat up a pan with the oil over medium heat, add the chard, tomatoes and the other ingredients, toss, and cook for 20 minutes.
2. Divide everything between plates and serve.

Nutrition:

calories 140, fat 4, fiber 2, carbs 4, protein 18

Mustard and Thyme Lamb Leg

Prep time: 5 minutes | **Cooking time:** 8 hours

Servings: 2

Ingredients:

- 1 pound lamb leg
- A pinch of salt and black pepper
- 2 tablespoons mustard
- 1 tablespoon olive oil
- 1 tablespoon thyme, chopped
- 2 garlic cloves, minced
- ½ cup beef stock
- 1 tablespoon chives, chopped

Directions:

1. In a slow cooker, combine the lamb with the mustard, oil and the other ingredients, toss, put the lid on and cook on Low for 8 hours.
2. Divide everything between plates and serve.

Nutrition:

calories 400, fat 34, fiber 1, carbs 3, protein 26

Ketogenic Dessert Recipes

Cooking time: 15 minutes | Servings: 2

Ingredients:
- ¼ cup almond milk
- 1 cup heavy cream
- 1 tablespoon stevia
- 1 teaspoon vanilla extract
- 2 tablespoons ghee, melted
- 2 eggs

Directions:
1. In a bowl, combine the cream with the milk and the other ingredients, whisk and divide into 2 ramekins.
2. Introduce the ramekins in the oven at 350 degrees F and bake for 15 minutes.
3. Serve warm.

Nutrition: calories 457, fat 46.5, fiber 0.7, carbs 3.9, protein 7.5

Stevia Cream

Prep time: 10 minutes | Cooking time: 20 minutes | Servings: 2

Ingredients:
- 2 tablespoons ghee, melted
- 1 cup coconut cream
- ½ cup coconut milk
- 1 tablespoon walnuts, chopped
- 1 tablespoon stevia
- ¼ cup coconut flesh, unsweetened and shredded

Directions:
1. In a bowl, combine ghee with the cream and the other ingredients, whisk well and divide into 2 ramekins.
2. Bake at 360 degrees F for 20 minutes and serve warm.

Nutrition: calories 550, fat 57.9, fiber 4.2, carbs 10.4, protein 5.1

Heavy Cream Mix

Prep time: 10 minutes | Cooking time: 20 minutes | Servings: 2

Ingredients:
- 1 cup heavy cream
- 1 tablespoon stevia
- 2 teaspoons cinnamon powder
- 2 eggs, whisked
- 1 teaspoon vanilla extract

Directions:
1. In a bowl, combine the cream with the stevia and the other ingredients, whisk and divide into 2 ramekins.
2. Cook at 390 degrees F for 20 minutes, cool down and serve.

Nutrition: calories 276, fat 26.5, fiber 0, carbs 2.4, protein 6.8

Berries Mix

Prep time: 10 minutes | Cooking time: 20 minutes | Servings: 2

Ingredients:
- 1 cup coconut cream
- 1 cup blackberries
- ½ cup blueberries
- 1 tablespoon swerve
- ½ teaspoon vanilla extract

Directions:
1. In a bowl, combine the cream with the berries and the other ingredients, transfer to a ramekin, and cook at 350 degrees F for 20 minutes.
2. Divide into bowls and serve.

Nutrition: calories 331, fat 29.1, fiber 7.3, carbs 19, protein 4

Ginger Bowls

Prep time: 5 minutes | Servings: 2

Ingredients:
- 2 tablespoons swerve
- 1 cup avocado, peeled, pitted and cubed
- 1 tablespoon ginger, grated
- Juice of ½ lime
- ½ teaspoon vanilla extract

Directions:
1. In a bowl, combine the avocado with the ginger and the other ingredients, toss and serve cold.

Nutrition: calories 244, fat 25.4, fiber 1.3, carbs 5.2, protein 2

Ginger Cookies

Prep time: 10 minutes | Cooking time: 20 minutes | Servings: 2

Ingredients:
- ½ cup almonds, chopped
- 2 eggs, whisked
- 3 tablespoons ghee, melted
- ½ cup coconut cream
- 2 tablespoons stevia
- ½ teaspoon ginger, ground
- 1 teaspoon baking powder

Directions:
1. In a blender, combine the almonds with the eggs and the other ingredients, whisk, take spoonfuls of this mix, arrange them on a lined baking sheet, flatten them a bit and cook at 360 degrees F for 20 minutes.
2. Serve the cookies cold.

Nutrition: calories 452, fat 41.6, fiber 6.5, carbs 11.7, protein 19

Swerve and Watermelon Mix

Prep time: 10 minutes | Servings: 2

Ingredients:
- 1 cup watermelon, peeled and cubed
- 2 tablespoons almonds, chopped
- ½ cup walnuts, chopped
- 1 tablespoon swerve
- 1 tablespoon lime juice

Directions:
1. In a bowl, combine the watermelon with the almonds, walnuts and the other ingredients, toss and serve.

Nutrition: calories 223, fat 32, fiber 1, carbs 3, protein 6

Ghee and Mint Cookies

Prep time: 10 minutes | Cooking time: 20 minutes | Servings: 2

Ingredients:
- ¼ cup coconut flour
- 2 eggs, whisked
- 2 tablespoons ginger, grated
- 1 tablespoon mint, chopped
- ½ cup coconut cream
- 3 tablespoons ghee, melted
- 3 tablespoons stevia
- 2 teaspoons baking powder

Directions:
1. In a bowl, combine the eggs with the flour and the other ingredients and whisk well.
2. Shape balls out of this mix, place them on a lined baking sheet, flatten them, introduce in the oven at 370 degrees F, bake for 20 minutes and serve them cold.

Nutrition: calories 190, fat 7.32, fiber 2.2, carbs 4, protein 3

Vanilla and Berries Bowls

Prep time: 5 minutes | **Servings:** 2

Ingredients:
- 1 tablespoon swerve
- 1 cup blackberries
- ½ cup strawberries
- 2 tablespoons almonds
- 1 teaspoon vanilla extract
- Zest of ½ lime, grated

Directions:
1. In a bowl, combine the berries with the almonds and the other ingredients, toss, divide into smaller bowls and serve.

Nutrition:
calories 140, fat 2, fiber 2, carbs 4, protein 4

Plums Mix

Prep time: 5 minutes | **Servings:** 2

Ingredients:
- 2 tablespoons swerve
- 1 cup plums, pitted and halved
- Juice of 1 lime
- ½ cup coconut cream

Directions:
1. In a bowl, combine the plums with the cream, stevia and the lime juice, toss and serve.

Nutrition:
calories 400, fat 23, fiber 4, carbs 6, protein 7

Plum and Vanilla Bowls

Prep time: 5 minutes | **Servings:** 2

Ingredients:
- 2 avocados, pitted, peeled and cubed
- 1 cup plums, pitted and halved
- ½ teaspoon vanilla extract
- Juice of 1 lime
- 1 tablespoon stevia

Directions:
1. In a bowl, combine the avocados with the plums and the other ingredients, toss and serve.

Nutrition:
calories 150, fat 3, fiber 3, carbs 5, protein 6

Mint and Watermelon Salad

Prep time: 10 minutes | **Servings:** 4

Ingredients:
- 1 cup watermelon, peeled and cubed
- 1 cup blackberries
- 1 tablespoon stevia
- 1 tablespoon lemon juice
- 1 tablespoon mint, chopped

Directions:
1. In a bowl, combine the berries with the watermelon and the other ingredients, toss and serve.

Nutrition:
calories 271, fat 24.5, fiber 6.3, carbs 14.1, protein 2.8

Lime Mousse

Prep time: 10 minutes | **Servings:** 2

Ingredients:
- 2 cups heavy cream
- Zest of 1 lime, grated
- 1 tablespoon cocoa powder
- 1 teaspoon vanilla extract
- 1 tablespoon stevia

Directions:
1. In a blender, combine the cocoa with the cream and the other ingredients, pulse well, divide into bowls and serve cold.

Nutrition:
calories 219, fat 21.1, fiber 0.9, carbs 7, protein 1.4

Coconut and Lime Zest Custard

Prep time: 10 minutes | **Cooking time:** 20 minutes | **Servings:** 2

Ingredients:
- 1 tablespoon stevia
- ½ tablespoon lime zest, grated
- 1 cup coconut milk
- 1 cup coconut cream
- ½ teaspoon vanilla extract
- 1 teaspoon cinnamon powder

Directions:
1. In a pan, combine the cream with the milk and the other ingredients, whisk, cook for 20 minutes over medium heat, divide into bowls and serve cold.

Nutrition:
calories 200, fat 2, fiber 1, carbs 3, protein 5

Aromatic Blueberries Mousse

Prep time: 10 minutes | **Servings:** 2

Ingredients:
- 1 cup coconut cream
- ½ cup avocado, peeled, pitted and cubed
- 1 cup blueberries
- ¾ teaspoon vanilla/stevia

Directions:
1. In a blender, combine the cream with the berries and the other ingredients, pulse well, divide into 2 bowls and serve.

Nutrition:
calories 143, fat 12, fiber 1, carbs 3, protein 2

Berries and Nutmeg Cream

Prep time: 2 hours | **Servings:** 2

Ingredients:
- 1 teaspoon nutmeg, ground
- ½ teaspoon vanilla extract
- 2 cups heavy cream
- ½ cup blackberries

Directions:
1. In a blender, combine the berries with the cream and the other ingredients, whisk and keep in the fridge for 2 hours before serving.

Nutrition:
calories 243, fat 22, fiber 0, carbs 6.2, protein 4

Walnuts and Avocado Bowls

Prep time: 10 minutes | **Servings:** 2

Ingredients:
- 1 cup walnuts
- ½ teaspoon stevia
- 1 avocado, peeled, pitted and cubed
- Juice of 1 lime
- ½ cup coconut cream

Directions:
1. In a bowl, combine the walnuts with the avocado and the other ingredients, whisk, divide into bowls and serve.

Nutrition:
calories 265, fat 6.3, fiber 2, carbs 4, protein 6

Cream Cheese Cream

Prep time: 10 minutes | **Servings:** 2

Ingredients:
- 1 cup coconut cream
- 1 tablespoon lime juice
- 1 tablespoon lime zest, grated
- 1 cup cream cheese
- ½ teaspoon vanilla extract

Directions:
1. In a blender, combine the cream with the lime juice and the other ingredients, whisk well, divide into bowls and serve cold.

Nutrition:
calories 332, fat 31.4, fiber 0.5, carbs 9.2, protein 5.5

Chia and Coconut Milk Pudding

Prep time: 10 minutes | **Cooking time:** 15 minutes | **Servings:** 2

Ingredients:
- 2 tablespoons ghee, melted
- 1 cup coconut milk
- ½ teaspoon baking soda
- 3 tablespoons chia seeds
- ½ teaspoon vanilla extract

Directions:
1. Heat up a pot with the ghee over medium heat, add the milk, chia and the other ingredients, whisk, cook for 15 minutes, divide into bowls and serve.

Nutrition: calories 220, fat 2, fiber 0.5, carbs 2, protein 4

Watermelon Soup

Prep time: 15 minutes | **Servings:** 2

Ingredients:
- 1 cup watermelon, peeled and cubed
- 1 tablespoon lime juice
- 1 teaspoon vanilla extract
- 2 tablespoons stevia

Directions:
1. In a blender, combine the watermelon with the vanilla and the other ingredients, pulse well, divide into bowls and serve.

Nutrition: calories 178, fat 4.4, fiber 2, carbs 3, protein 5

Cherries and Ginger Bowls

Prep time: 10 minutes | **Cooking time:** 10 minutes | **Servings:** 2

Ingredients:
- 1 cup cherries, pitted
- ½ teaspoon vanilla extract
- 2 tablespoons stevia
- ½ teaspoon ginger, ground
- 1 cup water
- Juice of ½ lime

Directions:
1. Heat up a pan with the water over medium heat, add the cherries, stevia and the other ingredients, toss, cook for 10 minutes, divide into bowls and serve.

Nutrition: calories 176, fat 15, fiber 2, carbs 5, protein 3

Green Tea Drink

Prep time: 5 minutes | **Servings:** 2

Ingredients:
- ½ cup almond milk
- 2 teaspoons lime zest
- 2 tablespoons green tea powder
- 1 tablespoon lime juice
- 1 tablespoon stevia

Directions:
1. In a blender, combine the almond milk with the green tea powder and the other ingredients, pulse well, divide into 2 glasses and serve.

Nutrition: calories 87, fat 5, fiber 3, carbs 6, protein 8

Lime and Stevia Mix

Prep time: 10 minutes | **Servings:** 2

Ingredients:
- 1 cup avocado, peeled, pitted and cubed
- Juice of 1 lime
- Zest of ½ lime, grated
- 1 cup coconut milk
- 1 teaspoon lemon stevia

Directions:
1. In a blender, combine the avocado with the milk and the other ingredients, pulse well, divide into bowls and serve cold.

Nutrition: calories 425, fat 42.9, fiber 7.5, carbs 12.9, protein 4.1

Vanilla Fudge

Prep time: 2 hours | **Cooking time:** 10 minutes | **Servings:** 2

Ingredients:
- ½ cup ghee, soft
- 2 teaspoons vanilla stevia
- ¼ cup coconut milk
- ½ teaspoon vanilla extract
- 1 tablespoon coconut oil

Directions:
1. In a pan, combine the ghee with the coconut milk, vanilla and the other ingredients, whisk, cook for 10 minutes over medium heat, transfer to a square pan, keep in the fridge for 2 hours, slice and serve.

Nutrition: calories 265, fat 23, fiber 2, carbs 4, protein 6

Berry Stew

Prep time: 10 minutes | **Cooking time:** 20 minutes | **Servings:** 2

Ingredients:
- 1 cup raspberries
- ½ teaspoon vanilla extract
- 1 cup water
- 3 tablespoons stevia
- Juice of 1 lime

Directions:
1. In a pan, combine the raspberries with the water, stevia and the other ingredients, whisk, cook over medium heat for 20 minutes, divide into bowls and serve really cold.

Nutrition: calories 60, fat 0, fiber 0, carbs 0, protein 2

Delicious Keto Smoothie

Prep time: 10 minutes | **Servings:** 2

Ingredients:
- ½ cup raspberries
- 1 cup almond milk
- 1 cup avocado, peeled, pitted and cubed
- ½ tablespoon stevia
- 1 tablespoon lemon juice

Directions:
1. In a blender, combine the raspberries with the avocado and the other ingredients, pulse well, divide into 2 glasses and serve.

Nutrition: calories 234, fat 22, fiber 2, carbs 4, protein 2

Coconut and Cinnamon Bars

Prep time: 10 minutes | **Cooking time:** 20 minutes | **Servings:** 2

Ingredients:
- 1 tablespoon ghee, melted
- ¼ cup coconut, unsweetened and shredded
- ½ teaspoon baking powder
- 2 tablespoons swerve
- ½ cup cream cheese
- 1 teaspoon cinnamon powder
- 2 eggs, whisked

Directions:
1. In a blender, combine the ghee with the baking powder, swerve and the other ingredients, pulse well and spread into a square baking dish.
2. Bake at 350 degrees F for 20 minutes, cut into bars and serve.

Nutrition: calories 358, fat 34.3, fiber 0.9, carbs 4, protein 10.3

Cocoa and Chia Bowl

Prep time: 15 minutes | **Servings:** 2

Ingredients:

- 1 cup coconut milk
- 2 tablespoons chia seeds
- 4 tablespoons cocoa powder
- 1 teaspoon vanilla extract
- 1 tablespoon almonds, chopped

Directions:

1. In a bowl, combine the milk with the chia seeds and the other ingredients, whisk, divide into smaller bowls, leave aside for 15 minutes and serve.

Nutrition:

calories 100, fat 10, fiber 1, carbs 3, protein 2

Berry Pie

Prep time: 2 minutes | **Cooking time:** 25 minutes | **Servings:** 2

Ingredients:

- 4 tablespoons coconut flour
- 2 tablespoon coconut oil, melted
- 2 teaspoons stevia
- ½ teaspoon vanilla extract
- 1 cup blackberries
- 2 eggs, whisked
- ½ teaspoon baking powder

Directions:

1. In a bowl, combine the flour with the oil, berries and the other ingredients, whisk well, divide into 2 ramekins and cook at 370 degrees F for 25 minutes.
2. Serve the cakes cold.

Nutrition:

calories 450, fat 34, fiber 7, carbs 10, protein 20

Almond and Rice Pudding

Prep time: 10 minutes | **Cooking time:** 20 minutes | **Servings:** 2

Ingredients:

- ½ cup blueberries
- 1 cup cauliflower rice
- 2 cups almond milk
- 2 tablespoons swerve
- 1 teaspoon vanilla extract

Directions:

1. In a pan, combine the rice with the milk and the other ingredients, toss, bring to a simmer and cook over medium heat for 20 minutes.
2. Divide into bowls and serve.

Nutrition:

calories 100, fat 3, fiber 3, carbs 6, protein 6

Watermelon Custard

Prep time: 10 minutes | **Cooking time:** 30 minutes | **Servings:** 2

Ingredients:

- 1 cup almond milk
- 1 cup watermelon, peeled and cubed
- 2 eggs
- 2 tablespoons swerve
- 2 tablespoons lemon juice

Directions:

1. In a blender, combine the watermelon with the milk and the other ingredients, pulse, divide into 2 ramekins and bake in the oven at 360 degrees F for 30 minutes.
2. Leave the custard to cool down before serving.

Nutrition:

calories 120, fat 6, fiber 2, carbs 5, protein 7

Cinnamon Pudding

Prep time: 5 minute | **Cooking time:** 20 minutes | **Servings:** 2

Ingredients:

- ½ cup heavy cream
- 2 tablespoons cocoa powder
- 1 tablespoon stevia
- ½ teaspoon cinnamon powder
- ½ teaspoon baking powder
- 2 eggs, whisked

Directions:

1. In a bowl, combine the cream with the cocoa powder and the other ingredients, whisk, divide into 2 ramekins and cook at 370 degrees F for 20 minutes.
2. Serve the pudding cold.

Nutrition:

calories 78, fat 1, fiber 1, carbs 2, protein 0

Blackberries Salad

Prep time: 10 minutes | **Servings:** 2

Ingredients:

- ½ cup avocado, peeled, pitted and cubed
- ½ cup plums, stoned and cubed
- 1 cup blackberries
- 1 cup raspberries
- 2 tablespoons stevia
- ½ tablespoon lemon juice

Directions:

1. In a bowl, combine the avocado with the berries and the other ingredients, toss and serve.

Nutrition:

calories 245, fat 34, fiber 2, carbs 6, protein 2

Cauliflower Pudding

Prep time: 10 minutes | **Cooking time:** 20 minutes | **Servings:** 2

Ingredients:

- 1 cup coconut cream
- ½ cup coconut milk
- 1 cup cauliflower rice
- ½ teaspoon sweet paprika
- ½ teaspoon lime zest, grated

Directions:

1. In a pan, combine the milk with the cream, rice and the other ingredients, whisk, cook over medium heat for 20 minutes, divide into bowls and serve.

Nutrition:

calories 150, fat 12, fiber 2, carbs 6, protein 1

Coconut and Cocoa Balls

Prep time: 10 minutes | **Cooking time:** 10 minutes | **Servings:** 2

Ingredients:

- 1 tablespoon stevia
- 2 eggs, whisked
- ½ teaspoon ginger, ground
- ½ teaspoon cocoa powder
- 2 cup coconut, shredded and unsweetened
- 1 teaspoon vanilla extract

Directions:

1. In a bowl, combine the eggs with the stevia and the other ingredients and whisk well.
2. Shape small balls, place them on a lined baking sheet, and cook at 350 degrees F for 15 minutes.
3. Serve the balls cold.

Nutrition:

calories 55, fat 6, fiber 1, carbs 2, protein 1

Strawberry and Lime Saute

Prep time: 10 minutes | **Cooking time:** 20 minutes | **Servings:** 2

Ingredients:
- 1 tablespoon stevia
- 1 cup strawberries, halved
- 1 cup water
- Zest of 1 lime, grated
- Juice of 1 lime

Directions:
1. Heat up a small pan with the water over medium heat, add the strawberries and the other ingredients, toss, cook for 20 minutes, cool down, divide into bowls and serve.

Nutrition:
calories 300, fat 23, fiber 2, carbs 5, protein 7

Lime Mix

Prep time: 10 minutes | **Cooking time:** 12 minutes | **Servings:** 2

Ingredients:
- 1 cup coconut cream
- 2 teaspoons stevia
- ½ cup coconut, unsweetened and shredded
- 1 tablespoon lime juice
- ½ teaspoon vanilla extract

Directions:
1. In a pan, combine the cream with the coconut and the other ingredients, whisk, cook over medium heat for 12 minutes, divide into bowls and serve.

Nutrition:
calories 245, fat 24, fiber 1, carbs 5, protein 4

Cream Cheese Pudding

Prep time: 10 minutes | **Cooking time:** 30 minutes | **Servings:** 2

Ingredients:
- 1 teaspoon vanilla extract
- 1 cup almond milk
- 2 ounces cream cheese
- 2 eggs, whisked
- 1 tablespoon ghee, melted
- 1 tablespoon stevia

Directions:
1. In your blender, combine the almond milk with the cream cheese and the other ingredients, and pulse well.
2. Pour this into 2 greased ramekins, introduce in the oven at 350 degrees F, bake for 30 minutes and serve cold.

Nutrition:
calories 254, fat 24, fiber 1, carbs 2, protein 8

Cinnamon and Vanilla Balls

Prep time: 10 minutes | **Servings:** 2

Ingredients:
- 3 tablespoons ghee, melted
- 2 tablespoons almond flour
- 1 tablespoon coconut milk
- 1 teaspoon cinnamon, powder
- 2 teaspoons stevia
- ½ teaspoon vanilla extract

Directions:
1. In a bowl, mix the ghee with the almond flour and the other ingredients except the cinnamon, stir well and shape balls out of this mix.
2. Roll balls in cinnamon and keep them in the fridge until you serve.

Nutrition:
calories 89, fat 1, fiber 2, carbs 4, protein 2

Keto Cocoa Cream

Prep time: 10 minutes | **Cooking time:** 20 minutes | **Servings:** 2

Ingredients:
- 2 tablespoons cocoa powder
- 1 cup heavy cream
- ½ cup blackberries
- 1 tablespoon stevia

Directions:
1. In a blender, combine the cream with the cocoa and the other ingredients, pulse well, divide into 2 ramekins and bake at 390 degrees F for 20 minutes.
2. Serve cold.

Nutrition:
calories 234, fat 23.1, fiber 3.5, carbs 8.1, protein 2.7

Almond Cream

Prep time: 10 minutes**Nutmeg Cream**

Prep time: 10 minutes | **Cooking time:** 15 minutes | **Servings:** 2

Ingredients:
- 1 teaspoon nutmeg, ground
- ½ teaspoon vanilla extract
- 3 tablespoons ghee, melted
- 1 cup coconut cream
- ½ tablespoon stevia

Directions:
1. In a bowl, combine the ghee with the cream and the other ingredients, whisk well, divide into 2 ramekins, bake at 350 degrees F for 15 minutes, cool down and serve.

Nutrition:
calories 453, fat 48.1, fiber 2.9, carbs 7.3, protein 2.9

Blueberries Mousse

Prep time: 10 minutes | **Cooking time:** 15 minutes | **Servings:** 2

Ingredients:
- 1 cup almond milk
- 1 cup blueberries
- 2 tablespoons stevia
- 2 eggs, whisked
- ½ teaspoon baking powder
- ½ teaspoon vanilla extract

Directions:
1. In a blender, combine the berries with the almond milk and the other ingredients, whisk, divide into 2 ramekins and bake in the oven at 360 degrees F for 15 minutes.
2. Cool down and serve.

Nutrition:
calories 393, fat 37.3, fiber 9.1, carbs 16.9, protein 4.2

Sweet Cauli Rice

Prep time: 10 minutes | **Cooking time:** 20 minutes | **Servings:** 2

Ingredients:
- 1 teaspoon vanilla extract
- 2 tablespoons ghee, melted
- 1 cup cauliflower rice
- 2 cups almond milk
- 2 tablespoons swerve
- ½ teaspoon cinnamon powder

Directions:
1. Heat up a pot with the ghee over medium heat, add the rice, milk and the other ingredients, whisk and cook for 20 minutes.
2. Divide into bowls and serve.

Nutrition:
calories 230, fat 12.2, fiber 4.2, carbs 5.4, protein 5.8

Avocado and Vanilla Cakes

Prep time: 10 minutes | **Cooking time:** 25 minutes | **Servings:** 2

Ingredients:

- 2 eggs, whisked
- ½ cup avocado, peeled, pitted and cubed
- 1 teaspoon vanilla extract
- 1 cup almond flour
- 2 tablespoons stevia
- ½ cup coconut cream
- ½ cup cream cheese
- ½ teaspoon baking soda

Directions:

1. In your food processor, combine the eggs with the avocado and the rest of the ingredients, whisk well and divide into 2 ramekins.
2. Cook at 365 degrees F for 25 minutes, cool down and serve.

Nutrition:

calories 200, fat 13, fiber 2, carbs 5, protein 8

Coffee Mousse

Prep time: 10 minutes | **Cooking time:** 20 minutes | **Servings:** 2

Ingredients:

- ½ cup coffee, brewed
- ½ cup coconut cream
- 1 teaspoon vanilla extract
- 1 teaspoon espresso powder
- 1 teaspoon vanilla stevia

Directions:

1. 1. In a pan, combine the coffee with the cream and the other ingredients, whisk, cook over medium heat for 20 minutes, divide into bowls and serve.

Nutrition:

calories 160, fat 13, fiber 0, carbs 2, protein 7

Zucchini Mousse

Prep time: 10 minutes | **Cooking time:** 20 minutes | **Servings:** 2

Ingredients:

- ½ cup zucchinis, grated
- 1 cup cauliflower rice
- 2 cups almond milk, unsweetened
- 1 teaspoon vanilla extract
- 2 tablespoons ghee, melted
- 2 teaspoons stevia

Directions:

1. In a pan, combine the zucchinis with the rice, milk and the other ingredients, whisk, cook over medium heat for 20 minutes, divide into bowls and serve.

Nutrition:

calories 120, fat 1, fiber 2, carbs 4, protein 2

Avocado Mix

Prep time: 10 minutes | **Servings:** 2

Ingredients:

- 2 avocados, peeled, pitted and roughly cubed
- 1 teaspoon vanilla extract
- ½ tablespoon stevia
- 1 cup coconut cream
- Juice of ½ lime
- Zest of ½ lime, grated

Directions:

1. In a bowl, combine the avocados with the vanilla, stevia and the other ingredients, toss, divide into smaller bowls and serve.

Nutrition:

calories 692, fat 67.8, fiber 16.1, carbs 24.2, protein 6.6

Cherry and Lemon Cream

Prep time: 10 minutes | **Cooking time:** 14 minutes | **Servings:** 2

Ingredients:

- 1 cup cherries, pitted
- ½ teaspoon vanilla powder
- Zest of 1 lemon, grated
- 1 tablespoon lemon juice
- 1 cup coconut cream
- ½ tablespoon stevia

Directions:

1. 1. Heat up a pan with the cream over medium heat, add the cherries, vanilla and the other ingredients, whisk, cook for 14 minutes, blend using an immersion blender, divide into bowls and serve.

Nutrition:

calories 60, fat 1, fiber 1, carbs 2, protein 0.5

Sweet and Sour Mousse

Prep time: 10 minutes | **Cooking time:** 15 minutes | **Servings:** 2

Ingredients:

- 1 teaspoon gelatin
- 1 cup cream cheese
- 1 cup raspberries
- ½ cup coconut cream
- ½ tablespoon lemon juice
- ½ tablespoon stevia

Directions:

1. In a blender, combine the cream cheese with the gelatin and the other ingredients, pulse well, divide into 2 ramekins and cook at 350 degrees F for 15 minutes.
2. Serve the cream cold.

Nutrition:

calories 234, fat 23, fiber 2, carbs 6, protein 7

Nutmeg Berries Bowl

Prep time: 2 hours | **Cooking time:** 20 minutes | **Servings:** 2

Ingredients:

- 1 teaspoon vanilla extract
- 2 tablespoons ghee, melted
- 2 cups cream cheese, soft
- 1 cup raspberries
- 2 teaspoons granulated stevia
- 1 teaspoon nutmeg, ground

Directions:

1. In a blender, combine the ghee with the cream cheese and the other ingredients, pulse well and divide into 2 ramekins.
2. Cook at 370 degrees F for 20 minutes, and keep in the fridge for 2 hours before serving.

Nutrition:

calories 450, fat 43, fiber 3, carbs 7, protein 7

Keto Cheesecakes

Prep time: 10 minutes | **Cooking time:** 15 minutes | **Servings:** 2

Ingredients:

- 2 tablespoons ghee, melted
- 1 cup cream cheese, soft
- 2 eggs, whisked
- 2 tablespoons swerve
- 1 tablespoon cocoa powder
- 1/3 cup swerve

Directions:

1. In your blender, combine the ghee with the cream cheese and the other ingredients, pulse well, divide into 2 ramekins and cook at 350 degrees F for 15 minutes.
2. Serve the cheesecakes cold.

Nutrition:

calories 254, fat 23, fiber 0, carbs 1, protein 5

Seeds Mix

Prep time: 10 minutes | Servings: 2

Ingredients:

- 1 cup almonds
- 2 tablespoons stevia
- ½ cup pumpkin seeds
- ½ cup sunflower seeds
- 2 tablespoons ghee, melted
- 1 teaspoon vanilla extract

Directions:

1. In a bowl, combine the almonds with the stevia, seeds and the other ingredients, toss and serve.

Nutrition:

calories 120, fat 2, fiber 2, carbs 4, protein 7

Berries Saute

Prep time: 10 minutes | Cooking time: 15 minutes | Servings: 2

Ingredients:

- 2 tablespoons stevia
- 1 cup blackberries
- 1 cup blueberries
- 1 cup water
- Juice of ½ lime
- Zest of ½ lime, grated

Directions:

1. In a pan, combine the berries with the stevia and the other ingredients, toss, and cook over medium heat for 15 minutes.
2. Divide into bowls and serve cold.

Nutrition:

calories 40, fat 4.3, fiber 2.3, carbs 3.4, protein 0.8

Almond and Berries Muffins

Prep time: 10 minutes | Cooking time: 25 minutes | Servings: 2

Ingredients:

- 2 tablespoons ghee, melted
- 1 tablespoon stevia
- 1 cup strawberries, chopped
- ½ cup almond milk
- 2 eggs, whisked
- ¼ teaspoon vanilla extract
- 1 teaspoon baking powder

Directions:

1. In bowl, combine the ghee with the stevia, berries and the other ingredients, whisk well and divide into a lined muffin pan.
2. Bake at 370 degrees F for 25 minutes, cool down and serve.

Nutrition:

calories 344, fat 35.1, fiber 3.4, carbs 8.3, protein 4.5

Coconut Cream Cookies

Prep time: 10 minutes | Cooking time: 25 minutes | Servings: 2

Ingredients:

- 1 cup blueberries, mashed
- ½ cup coconut flour
- ½ cup coconut cream
- ½ teaspoon vanilla extract
- ½ teaspoon baking powder
- 2 tablespoons ghee, melted

Directions:

1. In a bowl, combine the berries with the flour, cream and the other ingredients, and whisk well.
2. 2Place spoonfuls of this mix on a lined baking sheet, cook at 370 degrees F for 25 minutes and serve cold.

Nutrition:

calories 150, fat 2, fiber 1, carbs 3, protein 6

Tender Avocado Pudding

Prep time: 10 minutes | Cooking time: 20 minutes | Servings: 2

Ingredients:

- 1 avocado, peeled, pitted and cubed
- 1 cup cauliflower rice
- 1 cup almond milk
- ½ tablespoon stevia
- ½ teaspoon vanilla extract
- ½ teaspoon ginger, ground

Directions:

1. Heat up a pan with the milk over medium heat, add the cauliflower rice and the other ingredients, toss, cook for 20 minutes, divide into bowls and serve.

Nutrition:

calories 140, fat 2, fiber 1, carbs 2, protein 4

Cocoa Powder Mix

Prep time: 2 hours | Servings: 2

Ingredients:

- 1 cup cream cheese
- 1 cup coconut cream
- 2 tablespoons cocoa powder
- 1 teaspoon cinnamon powder
- 1 tablespoon stevia
- 4 tablespoons almond milk

Directions:

1. In a blender, combine the cream with the cream cheese, cocoa and the other ingredients, pulse well, divide into bowls and keep in the fridge for 2 hours before serving.

Nutrition:

calories 200, fat 2, fiber 2, carbs 5, protein 5

Sweet and Sour Jam

Prep time: 5 minutes | Cooking time: 20 minutes | Servings: 2

Ingredients:

- Juice of 1 lemon
- Zest of 1 lemon, grated
- 1 cup water
- 3 tablespoons stevia

Directions :

1. In a pan, combine the lemon juice with the lemon zest and the other ingredients, stir, cook over medium heat for 20 minutes, blend a bit using an immersion blender, divide into bowls and serve cold.

Nutrition:

calories 67, fat 0, fiber 0, carbs 1, protein 1

Ghee Cupcakes

Prep time: 10 minutes | Cooking time: 25 minutes | Servings: 2

Ingredients:

- 2 tablespoons ghee, melted
- 1 tablespoon cocoa powder
- 1 tablespoon swerve
- ½ cup coconut cream
- ¼ teaspoon vanilla extract
- ¼ cup almond milk
- ½ teaspoon baking powder

Directions:

1. In a bowl, combine the ghee with the cocoa powder and the other ingredients, whisk well and divide into a cupcake pan.
2. Cook at 360 degrees F for 25 minutes and serve the cupcakes cold.

Nutrition:

calories 240, fat 23, fiber 4, carbs 5, protein 2

Recipe Index

A

almond
- Nuts Bowls, 10
- Almonds and Berries Bowls, 9
- Mix of Seeds Bowls, 26
- Avocado Smoothie, 10
- Coconut Cream Dip, 41
- Seeds and Nuts Snack, 37
- Shrimps with Almonds and Parmesan, 48
- Poultry and Spinach Mix, 63
- Vanilla and Berries Bowls, 84
- Swerve and Watermelon Mix, 83
- Ginger Cookies, 83
- Seeds Mix, 89
- Cocoa and Chia Bowl, 86

almond milk
- Green Spread, 14
- Almond and Vegetables Muffins, 24
- Vanilla Bowls, 8
- Cinnamon Bowls, 8
- Chia Pudding, 8
- Almond Pancakes, 17
- Turmeric Pancakes, 17
- Almond and Coconut Porridge Bowls, 21
- Morning Waffles, 25
- Avocado Smoothie, 10
- Tender Keto Muffins, 25
- Almond Cream, 87
- Almond and Berries Muffins, 89
- Blueberries Mousse, 87
- Sweet Cauli Rice, 87
- Almond and Rice Pudding, 86
- Watermelon Custard, 86
- Cream Cheese Pudding, 87
- Zucchini Mousse, 88
- Tender Avocado Pudding, 89
- Cocoa Powder Mix, 89
- Green Tea Drink, 85
- Delicious Keto Smoothie, 85
- Ghee Cupcakes, 89

artichoke
- Artichoke and Parmesan Spread, 49
- Rosemary Chicken with Artichokes, 55
- Chicken with Artichokes, 63
- Garam Masala Beef with Artichokes, 76
- Cheesy Artichokes, 69

arugula
- Hard Boiled Eggs Bowl, 11
- Arugula Salad, 27
- Salmon and Capers Salad, 20
- Keto Radish Salad, 13
- Lime Taste Salad, 29
- Keto Avocado Bowl, 29
- Baby Arugula Salad, 32
- Keto Eggs Salad, 43
- Tender Keto Salad, 74
- Cherry Tomatoes and Greens Salad, 69

asparagus
- Shrimps and Vegetables, 26
- Paprika Asparagus, 28
- Asparagus and Lime Zest Bowls, 42
- Asparagus and Tender Chicken Thighs, 62
- Pork Chops with Vegetables, 71
- Asparagus Stew, 69
- Garlic and Chives Asparagus, 68

avocado
- Green Avocado Salad, 9
- Black Olives Salad, 11
- Basil Salad, 21
- Stew Meat Bowls, 14
- Sweet Avocado Salad, 10
- Lime Juice and Poultry Salad, 21
- Almond and Coconut Porridge Bowls, 21
- Micro Greens Bowls, 10
- Mix of Seeds Bowls, 26
- Avocado and Eggs, 24
- Avocado Smoothie, 10
- Baby Spinach and Chicken Bowls, 21
- Capers and Tuna Salad, 18
- Baby Spinach and Avocado Salad, 17
- Cherry Tomatoes and Shrimps Bowl, 20
- Arugula Salad, 27
- Baby Spinach Soup, 21
- Kalamata and Chicken Salad, 25
- Garam Masala Meal, 15
- Rosemary Broccoli with Beef, 13
- Lemon Seabass with Avocado, 27
- Basil Salad, 28
- Cilantro and Vegetables Mix, 36
- Zucchini Medley, 30
- Keto Avocado Bowl, 29
- Dijon Mustard Mix, 35
- Greens and Capers Salad, 42
- Capers Salsa, 40
- Avocado Dip, 42
- Kale and Scallions Salsa, 37
- Rosemary Sea Bass, 49
- Avocado with Cod, 50
- Cauli and Shrimps, 48
- Avocado Mix with Calamari Rings, 47
- Zucchini and Ground Chicken Bowl, 57
- Herbs and Chicken Mix, 56
- Lemon Turkey Bowl, 59
- Cumin Pork with Avocado, 78
- Dill and Cayenne Pepper Beef, 72
- Cubed Avocado and Pork, 80
- Tender Keto Salad, 74
- Cilantro Avocado, 68
- Coconut Cream Zucchini, 70
- Chives and Avocado Mix, 66
- Cabbage and Scallions, 81
- Avocado Mix, 88
- Walnuts and Avocado Bowls, 84
- Plum and Vanilla Bowls, 84
- Ginger Bowls, 83
- Avocado and Vanilla Cakes, 88
- Blackberries Salad, 86
- Tender Avocado Pudding, 89
- Delicious Keto Smoothie, 85
- Lime and Stevia Mix, 85
- Aromatic Blueberries Mousse, 84
- Mint Spread, 40
- Rosemary Sprouts with Avocado, 81

avocado oil
- Hot Eggs, 18
- Basil Salad, 21
- Meat and Spinach Bowls, 16
- Onion Powder Eggs, 18
- Cheddar Cheese Bake, 18
- Chives, Spinach, and Shrimps, 11
- Cream and Cauliflower Soup, 19
- Tender Radish Stew, 31
- Cumin Green Beans, 34
- Dill and Cucumber Bowl, 32
- Scallions Dip, 44
- Olives and Cream Cheese Spread, 39
- Garlic Sea Bass, 38
- Cilantro Sea Bass, 41
- Sea Bass and Baby Kale Bowl, 53
- Oregano and Chili Cod, 49
- Coconut Cream Shrimps, 51
- Turmeric Calamari, 46
- Tender Sour Tuna, 51
- Nutmeg Salmon Bowl, 44
- Spiced Tuna Fillets, 53
- Cheese Chicken, 61
- Shredded Cabbage and Chicken Mix, 56
- Juicy Rosemary Pork, 66
- Cumin Pork with Avocado, 78
- Nutmeg Pork Cubes, 65
- Cubed Avocado and Pork, 80
- Italian Seasoning and Pesto Lamb, 73
- Chives Radishes, 68
- Turmeric Sliced Zucchini Mix, 74
- Garlic and Scallions Bok Choy, 82
- Broccoli Spread, 75

B

beans
- Basil and Shrimps Salad, 12
- Chili Pepper Soup, 25
- Turmeric Sprouts Soup, 19
- Walnuts and Beef Bowl, 17
- Green Beans with Chicken, 15
- Aromatic Keto Mix, 33
- Cumin Green Beans, 34
- Chives Stew, 36
- Classic Keto Bowl, 31
- Shrimps with Green Beans, 48
- Shrimps with Endives, 46
- Green Beans and Turkey, 58
- Green Beans with Chili Pork, 71
- Rosemary Green Beans, 80
- Basil Green Beans, 69

beef
- Meat and Spinach Bowls, 16
- Avocado and Eggs, 24
- Ground Beef Bowl, 23
- Ketogenic Lunch Recipes, 24
- Keto Vegetables and Beef Stew, 12
- Minced Garlic and Scallions Beef, 23
- Parsley Soup, 23
- Chili Powder Meat, 22
- Walnuts and Beef Bowl, 17
- Spiced Meat Stew, 16
- Aromatic Beef and Greens, 13
- Rosemary Broccoli with Beef, 13
- Soft Meatballs, 12
- Meat Muffins, 37
- Coconut Cream Beef, 76
- Cumin and Bell Pepper Pork, 67
- Chili Beef with Tarragon, 79
- Parmesan Meat, 65
- Kale and Ground Beef, 76
- Autumn Beef Mix, 65
- Tender Beef Stew Meat, 79

90 | The Keto for Two

Cheesy Cumin and Garlic Beef, 65
Garam Masala Beef with Artichokes, 76
Rosemary Beef with Swiss Chard, 78
Dill and Cayenne Pepper Beef, 72
Spicy Okra and Beef Bowl, 67
Succulent Beef, 81
Keto Meat with Vegetables, 67
Beef and Peppers, 66
Vinegar Beef, 72
Tender Beef Roast, 73

bell pepper
Garlic Shrimps Mix, 11
Meat and Spinach Bowls, 16
Cilantro Eggs, 26
Bell Peppers Scrambled Eggs, 26
Keto Passata, 11
Bell Peppers Saute, 26
White Mushrooms Stew, 23
Tender Tuna Mix, 13
Cumin Stew, 29
Rosemary Peppers, 32
Caraway Seeds Mix of Vegetables, 36
Peppers Salsa, 39
Dijon Shrimp Skewers, 43
Basil Tuna and Cayenne Pepper Bowl, 46
Shrimps and Bell Peppers Bowl, 52
Coriander Turkey Bowl, 55
Tender Chicken and Greens, 56
Poultry Stir Fry, 55
Cumin and Bell Pepper Pork, 67
Tender Beef Stew Meat, 79
Spicy Okra and Beef Bowl, 67
Beef and Peppers, 66
Tender Beef Roast, 73
Aromatic Parsley and Lamb Stew, 67
Tender Keto Salad, 74
Keto Broccoli Mix, 70
Garlic Peppers, 75

blackberries
Almonds and Berries Bowls, 9
Chia Pudding, 8
Blackberries Salad, 8
Micro Greens Bowls, 10
Keto Cocoa Cream, 87
Berries Mix, 83
Berries Saute, 89
Vanilla and Berries Bowls, 84
Berries and Nutmeg Cream, 84
Mint and Watermelon Salad, 84
Berry Pie, 86
Blackberries Salad, 86

blueberries
Blackberries Salad, 8
Berries Mix, 83
Berries Saute, 89
Blueberries Mousse, 87
Almond and Rice Pudding, 86
Coconut Cream Cookies, 89
Aromatic Blueberries Mousse, 84

bok choy
Turmeric Bok Choy, 76
Coconut Cream Bok Choy, 70
Paprika and Lime Bok Choy, 69
Garlic and Scallions Bok Choy, 82
Garlic Mushroom with Bok Choy, 66
Chives and Avocado Mix, 66

Creamy Sprouts, 79

broccoli
Green Spread, 14
Poultry Stew, 22
Passata Soup, 23
Rosemary Broccoli with Beef, 13
Salad with Lime Juice, 28
Indian Style Cauliflower, 33
Green Mushrooms, 32
Broccoli Bites, 39
Coconut Milk Cod, 50
Broccoli and Poultry Bowl, 60
Ketogenic Vegetable Recipes, 73
Broccoli Florets Bowl, 69
Keto Broccoli Mix, 70
Broccoli Spread, 75
Ginger and Rosemary Broccoli, 77

brussel sprouts
Turmeric Brussels Sprouts, 21
Turmeric Sprouts Soup, 19
Aromatic Brussel Sprouts, 34
Cilantro and Vegetables Mix, 36
Parsley and Shrimps Bowl, 43
Garlic Turkey Breast with Brussels Sprouts, 61
Cilantro Brussels Sprouts, 73
Garam Masala Brussels Sprouts, 75
Sprouts and Kale Bowl, 69
Rosemary Sprouts with Avocado, 81
Lemon and Coriander Brussels Sprouts, 80
Creamy Sprouts, 79
Fennel Mix, 79

C

cabbage
Cabbage Soup, 16
Radish and Cabbage, 28
Tender Red Cabbage, 32
Tender Fish and Cabbage Salad, 53
Shredded Cabbage and Chicken Mix, 56
Pork with Coriander and Shredded Cabbage, 67
Garam Masala Green Cabbage, 75
Cabbage and Scallions, 81

calamari
Turmeric Calamari, 46
Calamari with Zucchini Zoodles, 46
Green Onions Calamari, 50
Coriander Calamari with Olives, 49
Vegetables with Calamari, 51
Avocado Mix with Calamari Rings, 47

capers
Chicken Pan, 19
Capers Mix, 23
Salmon and Capers Salad, 20
Dill Zoodles, 29
Mustard Greens and Olives, 32
Greens and Capers Salad, 42
Capers Salsa, 40
Beef and Peppers, 66
Lamb with Capers, 74
Cubed Avocado and Pork, 80
Meat Salad with Capers, 72

cauliflower
Seafood and Parsley Bowls, 10
Cream and Cauliflower Soup, 19

Chives Cauliflower, 28
Lime and Vinegar Cauliflower, 30
Indian Style Cauliflower, 33
Rosemary Mushroom Rice, 33
Hot Cauli Rice, 32
Cayenne Pepper Cauli, 31
Chili Powder Salad, 35
Tender Ghee Rice, 35
Tender Zucchini Rice, 31
Vegetable Spread, 44
Cauli and Shrimps, 48
Cauliflower Florets with Ginger Chicken, 57
Pork and Cauli Mix, 66
Cumin Cauliflower, 77
Nutmeg Cauliflower, 80
Sweet Cauli Rice, 87
Almond and Rice Pudding, 86
Cauliflower Pudding, 86
Zucchini Mousse, 88
Tender Avocado Pudding, 89

celery
Chicken with Curry Paste and Coconut Cream, 55
Scallions and Celery Stalk Lamb, 71

cheese
Walnuts Dip, 38
Pesto and Zucchini Dip, 38
Radish Dip, 38
Lime Cream Dip, 39
Olives and Cream Cheese Spread, 39
Masala Dip, 39
Ghee and Garlic Spread, 40
Kale and Parsley Dip, 45
Poblano Peppers Dip, 40
Cucumber and Dill Dip, 42
Keto Vegetables Rolls, 43
Artichoke and Parmesan Spread, 49
Basil Pesto Dip, 41
Chili Dip, 54
Parsley Cheese Spread, 37
Mozzarella Chicken, 60
Cream Cheese Cream, 84
Avocado and Vanilla Cakes, 88
Cream Cheese Pudding, 87
Cocoa Powder Mix, 89
Sweet and Sour Mousse, 88
Nutmeg Berries Bowl, 88
Keto Cheesecakes, 88
Coconut and Cinnamon Bars, 85

cheese (cheddar)
Chives Muffins, 20
Keto Cheese Mix, 15
Oregano and Tuna Casserole, 14
Cheddar Cheese Bake, 18
Garlic Frittata, 26
Meat Casserole, 15
Cumin Green Beans, 34
Jalapeno and Cheddar Cheese Mix, 33
Cheese Dip, 45
Broccoli Bites, 39
Meat Muffins, 37
Tender Chicken Cubes with Kalamata Olives, 55
Cheddar Chicken Thighs, 58
Black Pepper Radishes, 70

Recipe Index | 91

cheese (mozzarella)
- Garlic Frittata, 26
- Cheese and Turkey Mix, 11
- Mozzarella Chicken, 60
- Poultry Bake, 62
- Seafood Meatballs, 45
- Cheese Sticks, 40
- Mozzarella and Vegetables Dip, 37
- Cheesy Cumin and Garlic Beef, 65

cheese (parmesan)
- Parmesan Eggs Mix, 14
- Parmesan Radishes, 34
- Kale and Parsley Dip, 45
- Cumin Bowls, 42
- Shrimps with Almonds and Parmesan, 48
- Cheese Chicken, 61
- Ghee and Parmesan Chicken, 60
- Parmesan Chicken with Radish, 59
- Parmesan Meat, 65
- Parmesan and Scallions Lamb Chops, 74
- Cheesy Artichokes, 69
- Artichoke and Parmesan Spread, 49

cherries
- Cherries and Ginger Bowls, 85
- Cherry and Lemon Cream, 88

chia seeds
- Cinnamon Bowls, 8
- Chia Pudding, 8
- Mix of Seeds Bowls, 26
- Chia and Flaxseeds Muffins, 47
- Chia and Coconut Milk Pudding, 85
- Cocoa and Chia Bowl, 86

chicken
- Parmesan Eggs Mix, 14
- Sweet Paprika Eggs Mix, 10
- Baby Spinach and Chicken Bowls, 21
- Poultry and Cucumber Salad, 18
- Chicken Pan, 19
- Keto Passata, 11
- Chicken Sauce, 19
- Spiced Chicken Pan, 19
- Jalapeno Chicken Thighs, 17
- Paprika Chicken Thighs, 25
- Kalamata and Chicken Salad, 25
- Green Beans with Chicken, 15
- Chicken Muffins, 45
- Spring Onions Chicken Bites, 40
- Garlic Wings, 42
- Turmeric Chicken, 55
- Cheese Chicken, 61
- Lime Zest Chicken, 62
- Chicken with Artichokes, 63
- Chili Chicken Wings, 64
- Spicy Chicken Breast Cubes, 60
- Cilantro Chicken, 63
- Garam Masala Chicken, 56
- Chicken and Leek Bowl, 64
- Chicken in Tender Sauce, 59
- Rosemary and Paprika Chicken, 62
- Zucchini and Ground Chicken Bowl, 57
- Shredded Cabbage and Chicken Mix, 56
- Tender Chicken Cubes with Kalamata Olives, 55
- Chicken with Curry Paste and Coconut Cream, 55
- Scallions Chicken Cubes, 61
- Tender Chicken and Greens, 56
- Herbs and Chicken Mix, 56
- Ghee and Parmesan Chicken, 60
- Coriander Chicken with Fennel, 57
- Basil and Garlic Chicken, 58
- Chives Chicken, 60
- Sesame and Ginger Chicken, 57
- Mozzarella Chicken, 60
- Mustard and Garlic Chicken, 58
- Chicken with Endives, 58
- Thyme Chicken, 64
- Mushrooms, Parsley, and Chicken Bowl, 60
- Hot Chicken, 64
- Parmesan Chicken with Radish, 59
- Green Beans and Turkey, 58
- Cheddar Chicken Thighs, 58
- Vegetables and Chicken Strips, 58
- Rosemary Chicken with Artichokes, 55
- Radish Halves with Chicken Cubes, 61
- Chicken Roast, 59
- Nutmeg Chicken Cubes, 61
- Cauliflower Florets with Ginger Chicken, 57
- Cumin and Coconut Cream Chicken Breast, 57
- Asparagus and Tender Chicken Thighs, 62

chard
- Rosemary Beef with Swiss Chard, 78
- Cilantro Swiss Chard, 80
- Cumin Swiss Chard with Kalamata Olives, 75
- Chard Bowl, 82
- Keto Broccoli Mix, 70

chives
- Scallions Eggs, 9
- White Mushroom and Cumin Eggs, 9
- Sweet Omelet, 21
- Dill Fritters, 14
- Chives Muffins, 20
- Ground Beef Bowl, 23
- Minced Garlic and Scallions Beef, 23
- Green Onions Shrimp, 25
- Cucumbers and Olives Salad, 27
- Turmeric Sprouts Soup, 19
- Chives Cauliflower, 28
- Flaked Red Pepper Mushrooms, 30
- Paprika Asparagus, 28
- Spring Onions Salad, 28
- Dill Mix, 35
- Cilantro and Vegetables Mix, 36
- Tarragon Fennel, 31
- Mustard Greens and Olives, 32
- Dijon Mustard Mix, 35
- Herbs de Provence Olives, 36
- Chives Stew, 36
- Cumin and Oregano Radish, 33
- Cayenne Pepper Cauli, 31
- Tender Ghee Rice, 35
- Oregano Dip, 37
- Cheese Dip, 45
- Pesto and Zucchini Dip, 38
- Masala Dip, 39
- Fish Platter, 45
- Chives Salsa, 42
- Sun Dried Tomatoes and Olives Salsa, 42
- Tender Lemon Shrimp, 38
- Tuna with Vegetables, 50
- Shrimps with Fresh Fennel Bulb, 46
- Aromatic Trout, 52
- Perfect Keto Tuna, 51
- Rosemary and Chives Salmon, 49
- Shrimps in Sauce, 48
- Lime Zest Chicken, 62
- Spicy Chicken Breast Cubes, 60
- Chili Powder Turkey, 63
- Basil and Garlic Chicken, 58
- Chives Chicken, 60
- Tender Turkey in Sauce, 62
- Hot Chicken, 64
- Green Beans and Turkey, 58
- Asparagus and Tender Chicken Thighs, 62
- Garlic Cubed Pork, 72
- Pork Chops with Vegetables, 71
- Rosemary Lamb, 77
- Nutmeg Pork Cubes, 65
- Garam Masala Beef with Artichokes, 76
- Mustard and Thyme Lamb Leg, 82
- Cumin Cauliflower, 77
- Keto Vegetables Stew, 82
- Tomato Passata Kale, 77
- Asparagus Stew, 69
- Garlic and Chives Asparagus, 68
- Chives Radishes, 68
- Basil Green Beans, 69
- Olives and Scallions Salad, 68
- Paprika and Lime Bok Choy, 69
- Chard Bowl, 82
- Chives and Avocado Mix, 66
- Fennel Mix, 79

coconut
- Nuts Bowls, 10
- Vanilla Bowls, 8
- Rosemary Porridge, 8
- Stevia and Nuts Bowls, 8
- Almond and Coconut Porridge Bowls, 21
- Spring Onions Dip, 44
- Thyme Chicken, 64
- Coconut and Cocoa Balls, 86
- Lime Mix, 87
- Coconut and Cinnamon Bars, 85

coconut cream
- Nuts Bowls, 10
- Sweet Avocado Salad, 10
- Almonds and Berries Bowls, 9
- Rosemary Porridge, 8
- Stevia and Nuts Bowls, 8
- Turmeric Pancakes, 17
- Almond and Coconut Porridge Bowls, 21
- Cheese and Turkey Mix, 11
- Cream and Cauliflower Soup, 19
- Garlic Zucchini, 17
- Baby Spinach Soup, 21
- Coconut Cream Soup, 12
- Tarragon Fennel, 31
- Caraway Seeds Mix of Vegetables, 36
- Coconut Cream and Cumin Radish Mix, 34
- Tender Ghee Rice, 35
- Oregano Dip, 37

Spring Onions Dip, 44
Green Dip, 41
Vegetable Spread, 44
Garlic Powder Dip, 44
Cheese Dip, 45
Lime Cream Dip, 39
Masala Dip, 39
Kale and Parsley Dip, 45
Mint Spread, 40
Chia and Flaxseeds Muffins, 47
Chili Dip, 54
Coconut Cream Dip, 41
Meat Muffins, 37
Mozzarella and Vegetables Dip, 37
Dijon Mustard Trout, 41
Coriander Cod, 50
Curry and Garlic Shrimps, 47
Chicken with Curry Paste and Coconut Cream, 55
Chives Chicken, 60
Mushrooms, Parsley, and Chicken Bowl, 60
Bella Mushrooms and Turkey, 59
Cumin and Coconut Cream Chicken Breast, 57
Coconut Cream Beef, 76
Coconut Aminos Pork, 78
Radish and Lamb Stew, 73
Cumin Cauliflower, 77
Coconut Cream Bok Choy, 70
Paprika and Lime Bok Choy, 69
Coconut Cream Zucchini, 70
Berries Mix, 83
Stevia Cream, 83
Avocado Mix, 88
Walnuts and Avocado Bowls, 84
Cream Cheese Cream, 84
Plums Mix, 84
Ghee and Mint Cookies, 83
Ginger Cookies, 83
Avocado and Vanilla Cakes, 88
Cauliflower Pudding, 86
Lime Mix, 87
Coconut and Lime Zest Custard, 84
Coffee Mousse, 88
Coconut Cream Cookies, 89
Cherry and Lemon Cream, 88
Cocoa Powder Mix, 89
Sweet and Sour Mousse, 88
Ghee Cupcakes, 89
Aromatic Blueberries Mousse, 84

coconut milk
Coconut Eggs, 10
Chives Muffins, 20
Curry Turkey, 22
Chicken Muffins, 45
Coconut Milk Cod, 50
Garam Masala Chicken, 56
Thyme Chicken, 64
Stevia Cream, 83
Chia and Coconut Milk Pudding, 85
Cocoa and Chia Bowl, 86
Cauliflower Pudding, 86
Cinnamon and Vanilla Balls, 87
Coconut and Lime Zest Custard, 84
Vanilla Fudge, 85

Lime and Stevia Mix, 85

cod
Parsley Fish Stew, 22
Garlic Mix, 15
Chili Cod, 48
Baked Cod with Parsley, 53
Coriander Cod, 50
Oregano and Chili Cod, 49
Avocado with Cod, 50
Cod with Coriander Sauce, 47
Coconut Milk Cod, 50

crab
Crab Mix, 20

cucumbers
Shallot Salad, 9
Baby Spinach and Chicken Bowls, 21
Poultry and Cucumber Salad, 18
Ketogenic Lunch Recipes, 24
Cucumbers and Olives Salad, 27
Baby Spinach Soup, 21
Salmon and Capers Salad, 20
Lunch Shrimps, 20
Marinated Cucumbers, 29
Sliced Cucumbers and Cabbage Salad, 29
Dill and Cucumber Bowl, 32
Chili Powder Salad, 35
Keto Salsa, 41
Cucumbers Salsa, 39
Chives Salsa, 42
Cucumber and Dill Dip, 42
Keto Vegetables Rolls, 43
Shrimps with Green Beans, 48
Rosemary and Chives Salmon, 49
Olives and Scallions Salad, 68
Ginger Smoothie, 10
Lime Taste Salad, 29

D
duck
Tender Duck, 64
Garam Masala Duck, 59

E
egg
Scallions Eggs, 9
Hard Boiled Eggs Bowl, 11
Red Pepper Flakes Eggs, 9
White Mushroom and Cumin Eggs, 9
Hot Eggs, 18
Turmeric Eggs with Shrimps, 20
Meat and Spinach Bowls, 16
Dill Fritters, 14
Oregano and Tuna Casserole, 14
Cilantro and Eggs Mix, 14
Coconut Eggs, 10
Salmon and Cumin Eggs, 9
Parmesan Eggs Mix, 14
Almond and Vegetables Muffins, 24
Onion Powder Eggs, 18
Ghee Eggs Mix, 21
Radish Hash, 8
Chives Muffins, 20
Kale Eggs, 8
Almond Pancakes, 17
Turmeric Pancakes, 17
Morning Waffles, 25
Sweet Paprika Eggs Mix, 10
Avocado and Eggs, 24

Green Lime Omelet, 18
Cilantro Eggs, 26
Garlic Frittata, 26
Bell Peppers Scrambled Eggs, 26
Cilantro Pork Meatballs, 12
Meat Casserole, 15
Coconut Muffins, 44
Chicken Muffins, 45
Seafood Meatballs, 45
Cheese Sticks, 40
Keto Eggs Salad, 43
Chia and Flaxseeds Muffins, 47
Meat Muffins, 37
Avocado and Vanilla Cakes, 88
Cinnamon Pudding, 86
Berry Pie, 86
Watermelon Custard, 86
Coconut and Cocoa Balls, 86
Keto Cheesecakes, 88
Sweet Omelet, 21
Cheddar Cheese Bake, 18
Tender Keto Muffins, 25
Soft Meatballs, 12
Almond Cream, 87
Heavy Cream Mix, 83
Almond and Berries Muffins, 89
Blueberries Mousse, 87
Ghee and Mint Cookies, 83
Ginger Cookies, 83
Cream Cheese Pudding, 87
Coconut and Cinnamon Bars, 85

endive
Turkey and Endives, 13
Fragrant Scallions, 32
Shrimps with Endives, 46
Trout Bowl, 49
Chicken with Endives, 58
Lime Juice Lamb Chops, 81
Oregano Endives, 82

F
fennel
Tarragon Fennel, 31
Fennel Bulb Salad, 29
Kalamata Olives and Fennel, 35
Shrimps with Fresh Fennel Bulb, 46
Coriander Chicken with Fennel, 57
Pork with Sliced Fennel, 74
Chili Fennel, 68
Fennel Mix, 79

G
garlic
Garlic Shrimps Mix, 11
Dill Fritters, 14
Radish Hash, 8
Kale Eggs, 8
Garlic Frittata, 26
Keto Passata, 11
Basil and Shrimps Salad, 12
Keto Vegetables and Beef Stew, 12
Chicken Sauce, 19
Minced Garlic and Scallions Beef, 23
Bell Peppers Saute, 26
Parsley Fish Stew, 22
Meat Casserole, 15
Garlic Mix, 15
Parsley Soup, 23

Recipe Index | 93

Chili Powder Meat, 22
Poultry Stew, 22
Curry Turkey, 22
Passata Soup, 23
Garlic Zucchini, 17
Turmeric Brussels Sprouts, 21
White Mushrooms Stew, 23
Aromatic Basil Shrimps, 22
Walnuts and Beef Bowl, 17
Spiced Meat Stew, 16
Vinegar Shrimps, 20
Kale and Garlic Soup, 16
Aromatic Beef and Greens, 13
Rosemary Broccoli with Beef, 13
Coconut Cream Soup, 12
Soft Meatballs, 12
Mushrooms and Pork, 13
Kale Saute, 28
Tender Radish Stew, 31
Aromatic Keto Mix, 33
Chives Cauliflower, 28
Cumin Kale, 34
Scallions Zucchini, 28
Aromatic Brussel Sprouts, 34
Fragrant Mushrooms, 34
Salad with Lime Juice, 28
Flaked Red Pepper Mushrooms, 30
Lime and Vinegar Cauliflower, 30
Parmesan Radishes, 34
Baby Spinach Saute, 29
Sliced Cucumbers and Cabbage Salad, 29
Dill Zoodles, 29
Green Chili Pepper Tomatoes, 30
Mustard Seeds Kale, 31
Dijon Mustard Mix, 35
Soft and Aromatic Radish Bowl, 33
Chives Stew, 36
Green Mushrooms, 32
Hot Cauli Rice, 32
Hemp Seeds Mushrooms, 30
Keto Caps, 35
Classic Keto Bowl, 31
Vegetable Spread, 44
Garlic Powder Dip, 44
Ghee and Garlic Spread, 40
Poblano Peppers Dip, 40
Lamb and Garlic Dip, 40
Garlic Wings, 42
Keto Crackers, 54
Dijon Shrimp Skewers, 43
Coconut Cream Dip, 41
Pesto Snack, 47
Parsley Cheese Spread, 37
Shrimps with Green Beans, 48
Coriander Cod, 50
Oregano and Chili Cod, 49
Curry and Garlic Shrimps, 47
Sour Cumin Shrimp, 47
Shrimps with Endives, 46
Mint and Garlic Shrimp, 54
Cod with Coriander Sauce, 47
Basil Tuna and Cayenne Pepper Bowl, 46
Coconut Cream Shrimps, 51
Shrimps and Bell Peppers Bowl, 52
Green Onions Calamari, 50
Red Pepper Flakes Trout, 48

Coriander Calamari with Olives, 49
Vegetables with Calamari, 51
Coconut Milk Cod, 50
Tarragon and Cumin Swordfish Steaks, 53
Marjoram Seafood Bowl, 52
Garlic Mussels, 53
Cilantro Chicken, 63
Garam Masala Chicken, 56
Garlic Turkey Breast with Brussels Sprouts, 61
Coriander Turkey Bowl, 55
Greens and Turkey Bowl, 62
Tender Chicken and Greens, 56
Leek and Turkey, 57
Coriander Chicken with Fennel, 57
Basil and Garlic Chicken, 58
Mustard and Garlic Chicken, 58
Thyme Chicken, 64
Mustard Powder Turkey, 64
Parmesan Chicken with Radish, 59
Radish Halves with Chicken Cubes, 61
Chicken Roast, 59
Aromatic Spiced Turkey, 61
Nutmeg Chicken Cubes, 61
Cauliflower Florets with Ginger Chicken, 57
Cumin and Coconut Cream Chicken Breast, 57
Juicy Rosemary Pork, 66
Garlic Cubed Pork, 72
Chili Powder Pork Stew Meat, 74
Coconut Cream Beef, 76
Cumin and Bell Pepper Pork, 67
Rosemary Pork Cubes, 78
Pork and Zucchini, 65
Kale and Ground Beef, 76
Autumn Beef Mix, 65
Cheesy Cumin and Garlic Beef, 65
Mint Lamb Cubes, 72
Chili and Chives Lamb, 71
Cumin and Chili Powder Lamb Chops, 76
Scallions and Celery Stalk Lamb, 71
Parsley Lamb Cubes, 72
Keto Lamb Bowl, 71
Mustard and Thyme Lamb Leg, 82
Tender Cilantro Lamb Chops, 75
Lime Juice Lamb Chops, 81
Spring Pork Stew, 67
Chili Lamb with Mushrooms, 78
Succulent Beef, 81
Lamb with Capers, 74
Soft Ghee Lamb, 82
Ketogenic Vegetable Recipes, 73
Keto Vegetables Stew, 82
Cilantro Swiss Chard, 80
Oregano Endives, 82
Rosemary Green Beans, 80
Nutmeg Cauliflower, 80
Garlic Okra, 81
Greens Bowl, 70
Garlic and Chives Asparagus, 68
Broccoli Florets Bowl, 69
Zucchini Cubes Stew, 69
Paprika and Lime Bok Choy, 69
Cumin Swiss Chard with Kalamata

Olives, 75
Garlic and Scallions Bok Choy, 82
Coconut Cream Zucchini, 70
Broccoli Spread, 75
Garlic Peppers, 75
Garlic Mushroom with Bok Choy, 66
Chives and Avocado Mix, 66
Lemon and Coriander Brussels Sprouts, 80
Creamy Sprouts, 79
Red Chili Baby Spinach, 80

ginger
Ginger Smoothie, 10
Poultry and Fish Soup, 16
Perfect Keto Tuna, 51
Ginger and Cumin Salmon, 51
Ginger Tuna, 43
Sesame and Ginger Chicken, 57
Mustard and Garlic Chicken, 58
Cauliflower Florets with Ginger Chicken, 57
Chili and Chives Lamb, 71
Ginger and Rosemary Broccoli, 77
Ghee and Mint Cookies, 83
Ginger Bowls, 83
Ginger Cookies, 83
Tender Avocado Pudding, 89

H
heavy cream
Garlic Peppers, 75
Creamy Sprouts, 79
Keto Cocoa Cream, 87
Almond Cream, 87
Heavy Cream Mix, 83
Lime Mousse, 84
Berries and Nutmeg Cream, 84
Cinnamon Pudding, 86
Mint Lamb Cubes, 72

K
kale
Shallot Salad, 9
Kale Eggs, 8
Blackberries Salad, 8
Avocado Smoothie, 10
Capers and Tuna Salad, 18
Lime Juice and Chives Salad, 24
Garlic Mix, 15
Kale and Garlic Soup, 16
Kale Saute, 28
Cumin Kale, 34
Mustard Seeds Kale, 31
Kale and Parsley Dip, 45
Keto Crackers, 54
Kale and Scallions Salsa, 37
Sea Bass and Baby Kale Bowl, 53
Vegetables and Chicken Strips, 58
Kale and Ground Beef, 76
Beef and Peppers, 66
Tomato Passata Kale, 77
Sprouts and Kale Bowl, 69
Baby Kale and Halved Radish, 70
Baby Kale Mix, 68
Sesame and Coriander Kale, 80

L
lamb

White Mushrooms and Lamb Mix, 27
Lamb and Garlic Dip, 40
Scallions Lamb Chops, 73
Garam Masala Lamb, 76
Rosemary Lamb, 77
Tender Lamb with Ghee, 65
Aromatic Lamb Chops, 79
Mint Lamb Cubes, 72
Chili Peppers Lamb Chops, 71
Chili and Chives Lamb, 71
Cumin and Chili Powder Lamb Chops, 76
Scallions and Celery Stalk Lamb, 71
Parsley Lamb Cubes, 72
Keto Lamb Bowl, 71
Lemon Lamb, 81
Mustard and Thyme Lamb Leg, 82
Tender Sour Lamb Riblets, 77
Tender Cilantro Lamb Chops, 75
Lime Juice Lamb Chops, 81
Parmesan and Scallions Lamb Chops, 74
Chili Lamb with Mushrooms, 78
Lamb with Capers, 74
Soft Ghee Lamb, 82
Coriander Meat Stew, 66
Italian Seasoning and Pesto Lamb, 73
Aromatic Parsley and Lamb Stew, 67
Radish and Lamb Stew, 73
Meat Salad with Capers, 72

leek
Cilantro and Eggs Mix, 14
Sweet Paprika Eggs Mix, 10
Ghee and Garlic Spread, 40
Chicken and Leek Bowl, 64
Leek and Turkey, 57
Tender Lamb with Ghee, 65
Keto Vegetables Stew, 82

lemon
Keto Radish Salad, 13
Parsley and Shrimps Bowl, 43
Coriander Calamari with Olives, 49
Lemon Turkey Bowl, 59
Lemon Lamb, 81
Succulent Beef, 81
Asparagus Stew, 69
Turmeric Sliced Zucchini Mix, 74
Lemon and Coriander Brussels Sprouts, 80
Cherry and Lemon Cream, 88
Sweet and Sour Jam, 89

lime
Spiralized Salad, 19
Chicken Sauce, 19
White Mushrooms and Lamb Mix, 27
Lunch Shrimps, 20
Basil Salad, 28
Salad with Lime Juice, 28
Paprika Asparagus, 28
Lime and Vinegar Cauliflower, 30
Sliced Cucumbers and Cabbage Salad, 29
Green Chili Pepper Tomatoes, 30
Cajun Seasonings and Keto Vegetables, 36
Chili Powder Salad, 35
Keto Salsa, 41
Walnuts Dip, 38
Lime Cream Dip, 39

Lime Cream Dip, 39
Nutmeg Platter, 40
Italian Style Shrimps, 45
Mint Spread, 40
Salmon Mix, 43
Asparagus and Lime Zest Bowls, 42
Lime Salmon, 38
Sour Cumin Shrimp, 47
Calamari with Zucchini Zoodles, 46
Fennel Seeds Shrimp, 43
Ginger Tuna, 43
Avocado Mix with Calamari Rings, 47
Trout Bowl, 49
Lime Zest Chicken, 62
Chili Peppers Lamb Chops, 71
Garlic Okra, 81
Baby Kale and Halved Radish, 70
Cilantro Avocado, 68
Avocado Mix, 88
Lime Mousse, 84
Cream Cheese Cream, 84
Strawberry and Lime Saute, 87
Green Tea Drink, 85
Lime and Stevia Mix, 85

M
mushrooms
Keto Caps, 35
Dill Fritters, 14
Rosemary Porridge, 8
Ground Beef Bowl, 23
Basil and Seafood Bowls, 16
Fragrant Mushrooms, 34
Flaked Red Pepper Mushrooms, 30
Green Mushrooms, 32
Rosemary Mushroom Rice, 33
Hemp Seeds Mushrooms, 30
Mushrooms, Parsley, and Chicken Bowl, 60
Keto Meat with Vegetables, 67
Coriander Meat Stew, 66
Garlic Mushroom with Bok Choy, 66

mushrooms (bella)
Bella Mushrooms and Turkey, 59
Chili Lamb with Mushrooms, 78

mushrooms (white)
White Mushroom and Cumin Eggs, 9
Spiralized Salad, 19
Baby Spinach and Avocado Salad, 17
White Mushrooms Stew, 23
White Mushrooms and Lamb Mix, 27
Coconut Cream Soup, 12

mussels
Garlic Mussels, 53

O
okra
Spicy Okra and Beef Bowl, 67
Keto Meat with Vegetables, 67
Aromatic Parsley and Lamb Stew, 67
Keto Vegetables Stew, 82
Garlic Okra, 81

olives
Black Olives Salad, 11
Lime Zest Salad, 9
Cucumbers and Olives Salad, 27
Salmon Stew, 15
Crab Mix, 20

Kalamata and Chicken Salad, 25
Garam Masala Meal, 15
Keto Style Mix, 12
Lime Taste Salad, 29
Dill Mix, 35
Zucchini Medley, 30
Keto Avocado Bowl, 29
Baby Arugula Salad, 32
Mustard Greens and Olives, 32
Kalamata Olives and Fennel, 35
Herbs de Provence Olives, 36
Soft and Aromatic Radish Bowl, 33
Hemp Seeds Mushrooms, 30
Keto Salsa, 41
Olives and Cream Cheese Spread, 39
Cucumbers Salsa, 39
Peppers Salsa, 39
Shrimp and Curry Powder Salsa, 45
Sun Dried Tomatoes and Olives Salsa, 42
Basil Pesto Dip, 41
Seeds and Nuts Snack, 37
Kale and Scallions Salsa, 37
Baby Spinach and Fish Salad, 46
Coriander Calamari with Olives, 49
Tender Fish and Cabbage Salad, 53
Chicken and Leek Bowl, 64
Tender Chicken Cubes with Kalamata Olives, 55
Tender Turkey in Sauce, 62
Rosemary Chicken with Artichokes, 55
Kale and Ground Beef, 76
Olives and Scallions Salad, 68
Spring Salad, 68
Cumin Swiss Chard with Kalamata Olives, 75
Dill Mix, 79

onion
Hard Boiled Eggs Bowl, 11
Red Pepper Flakes Eggs, 9
White Mushroom and Cumin Eggs, 9
Garlic Shrimps Mix, 11
Green Avocado Salad, 9
Turmeric Eggs with Shrimps, 20
Basil Salad, 21
Sweet Omelet, 21
Coconut Eggs, 10
Salmon and Cumin Eggs, 9
Almond and Vegetables Muffins, 24
Ghee Eggs Mix, 21
Capers and Tuna Salad, 18
Cheddar Cheese Bake, 18
Cilantro Eggs, 26
Garlic Frittata, 26
Ground Beef Bowl, 23
Tender Keto Muffins, 25
Chicken Pan, 19
Bell Peppers Scrambled Eggs, 26
Basil and Shrimps Salad, 12
Cherry Tomatoes and Shrimps Bowl, 20
Lime Juice and Chives Salad, 24
Green Onions Shrimp, 25
Garlic Mix, 15
Capers Mix, 23
Jalapeno Chicken Thighs, 17
Walnuts and Beef Bowl, 17
Spiced Meat Stew, 16

Recipe Index | 95

Tender Radish Stew, 31
Basil Salad, 28
Spring Onions Salad, 28
Spiced Vegetables, 30
Chives Stew, 36
Oregano Dip, 37
Scallions Dip, 44
Spring Onions Dip, 44
Chicken Muffins, 45
Cucumbers Salsa, 39
Spring Onions Chicken Bites, 40
Shrimp and Curry Powder Salsa, 45
Avocado Dip, 42
Chili Dip, 54
Ketogenic Seafood and Fish Recipes, 37
Shrimps with Chicken broth, 38
Rosemary Sea Bass, 49
Green Onions Calamari, 50
Balsamic Tuna with Spring Onions, 44
Nutmeg Salmon Bowl, 44
Tender Fish and Cabbage Salad, 53
Spiced Tuna Fillets, 53
Herbs and Chicken Mix, 56
Red Chili Pepper Turkey, 56
Garam Masala Duck, 59
Chicken Roast, 59
Nutmeg Pork Cubes, 65
Keto Lamb Bowl, 71
Vinegar Beef, 72
Cumin Cauliflower, 77
Tender Keto Salad, 74
Ginger and Rosemary Broccoli, 77
Lemon and Coriander Brussels Sprouts, 80

P

pepper (chili)
Garlic Sea Bass, 38
Avocado Mix with Calamari Rings, 47
Basil Cream, 70
Red Chili Baby Spinach, 80
Hot Eggs, 18
Spiced Chicken Pan, 19
Chili Pepper Soup, 25
Chili Powder Meat, 22
Mushrooms and Pork, 13
Green Chili Pepper Tomatoes, 30
Tender Red Cabbage, 32
Tender Zucchini Rice, 31
Oregano and Chili Cod, 49
Ginger Tuna, 43
Red Chili Pepper Turkey, 56
Chili Peppers Lamb Chops, 71
Mustard Seeds Kale, 31
Garlic Powder Dip, 44
Tender Salmon with Ghee, 51
Shrimps in Sauce, 48
Tender Duck, 64

pepper (jalapeno)
Jalapeno and Cheddar Cheese Mix, 33
Avocado Dip, 42
Parsley Cheese Spread, 37
Balsamic Tuna with Spring Onions, 44
Jalapeno Chicken Thighs, 17
Chives Salsa, 42
Hot Chicken, 64
Cheddar Chicken Thighs, 58

pine nuts
Fennel Bulb Salad, 29
Classic Keto Bowl, 31
Garlic Powder Dip, 44
Sun Dried Tomatoes and Olives Salsa, 42
Balsamic Tuna with Spring Onions, 44
Aromatic Shrimps with Pine Nuts, 50
Baby Spinach Bowl, 81

plums
Plums Mix, 84
Plum and Vanilla Bowls, 84
Blackberries Salad, 86

pork
Stew Meat Bowls, 14
Cilantro Pork Meatballs, 12
Meat Casserole, 15
Mushrooms and Pork, 13
Scallions Dip, 44
Juicy Rosemary Pork, 66
Garlic Cubed Pork, 72
Green Beans with Chili Pork, 71
Chili Powder Pork Stew Meat, 74
Pork Chops with Vegetables, 71
Cumin Pork Chops, 78
Cumin and Bell Pepper Pork, 67
Rosemary Pork Cubes, 78
Passata Pork Chops, 77
Cumin Pork with Avocado, 78
Pork and Zucchini, 65
Coconut Aminos Pork, 78
Pork with Sliced Fennel, 74
Nutmeg Pork Cubes, 65
Pork with Coriander and Shredded Cabbage, 67
Spring Pork Stew, 67
Pork and Cauli Mix, 66
Cubed Avocado and Pork, 80

R

radishes
Radish Hash, 8
Walnuts Salad, 27
Keto Radish Salad, 13
Tender Radish Stew, 31
Radish and Cabbage, 28
Cumin Kale, 34
Parmesan Radishes, 34
Spiced Vegetables, 30
Soft and Aromatic Radish Bowl, 33
Cumin and Oregano Radish, 33
Dill and Cucumber Bowl, 32
Coconut Cream and Cumin Radish Mix, 34
Radish Dip, 38
Cumin Bowls, 42
Vegetables with Calamari, 51
Vegetables with Calamari, 51
Parmesan Chicken with Radish, 59
Radish Halves with Chicken Cubes, 61
Radish and Lamb Stew, 73
Chives Radishes, 68
Black Pepper Radishes, 70
Baby Kale and Halved Radish, 70
Walnuts Salad, 74

raspberries
Spinach Bowl, 18
Blackberries Salad, 86

Berry Stew, 85
Sweet and Sour Mousse, 88
Nutmeg Berries Bowl, 88
Delicious Keto Smoothie, 85

S

salmon
Salmon Salad, 11
Salmon and Cumin Eggs, 9
Salmon Stew, 15
Salmon and Capers Salad, 20
Poultry and Fish Soup, 16
Garam Masala Meal, 15
Fish Platter, 45
Salmon Mix, 43
Ketogenic Seafood and Fish Recipes, 37
Lime Salmon, 38
Tender Salmon with Ghee, 51
Ginger and Cumin Salmon, 51
Rosemary and Chives Salmon, 49
Nutmeg Salmon Bowl, 44
Fish with Mustard Sauce, 52
Tender Fish and Cabbage Salad, 53
Salmon with Halved Tomatoes, 52

scallions
Scallions Eggs, 9
Scallions and Seafood Salad, 24
Stew Meat Bowls, 14
Oregano and Tuna Casserole, 14
Cilantro and Eggs Mix, 14
Green Spread, 14
Seafood and Parsley Bowls, 10
Allspice Zucchini, 24
Onion Powder Eggs, 18
Radish Hash, 8
Rosemary Porridge, 8
Sweet Paprika Eggs Mix, 10
Green Lime Omelet, 18
Cilantro Eggs, 26
Keto Passata, 11
Cilantro Pork Meatballs, 12
Keto Vegetables and Beef Stew, 12
Minced Garlic and Scallions Beef, 23
Bell Peppers Saute, 26
Salmon Stew, 15
Turkey Stew, 22
Cream and Cauliflower Soup, 19
Parsley Soup, 23
Poultry Stew, 22
Curry Turkey, 22
Passata Soup, 23
Garlic Zucchini, 17
White Mushrooms Stew, 23
Aromatic Basil Shrimps, 22
Turmeric Sprouts Soup, 19
Vinegar Shrimps, 20
Basil and Seafood Bowls, 16
Kale and Garlic Soup, 16
Poultry and Fish Soup, 16
Cabbage Soup, 16
Tender Tuna Mix, 13
Garam Masala Meal, 15
Aromatic Beef and Greens, 13
Soft Meatballs, 12
Mushrooms and Pork, 13
Keto Cheese Mix, 15
Turkey and Endives, 13

Radish and Cabbage, 28
Scallions Zucchini, 28
Flaked Red Pepper Mushrooms, 30
Baby Spinach Saute, 29
Marinated Cucumbers, 29
Spiced Vegetables, 30
Mustard Seeds Kale, 31
Fragrant Scallions, 32
Rosemary Peppers, 32
Tender Red Cabbage, 32
Kalamata Olives and Fennel, 35
Herbs de Provence Olives, 36
Jalapeno and Cheddar Cheese Mix, 33
Rosemary Mushroom Rice, 33
Hot Cauli Rice, 32
Coconut Cream and Cumin Radish Mix, 34
Cayenne Pepper Cauli, 31
Tender Ghee Rice, 35
Tender Zucchini Rice, 31
Scallions Dip, 44
Green Dip, 41
Cheese Dip, 45
Keto Eggs Salad, 43
Kale and Scallions Salsa, 37
Scallions Shrimps, 41
Dijon Mustard Trout, 41
Shrimps with Green Beans, 48
Sea Bass and Baby Kale Bowl, 53
Tuna with Vegetables, 50
Coriander Cod, 50
Aromatic Trout, 52
Coconut Cream Shrimps, 51
Turmeric Calamari, 46
Calamari with Zucchini Zoodles, 46
Thyme Seafood Bowl, 52
Fennel Seeds Shrimp, 43
Tender Sour Tuna, 51
Shrimps with Almonds and Parmesan, 48
Green Onions Calamari, 50
Fish with Mustard Sauce, 52
Salmon with Halved Tomatoes, 52
Garlic Mussels, 53
Turmeric Chicken, 55
Spicy Chicken Breast Cubes, 60
Garam Masala Chicken, 56
Oregano Turkey, 56
Broccoli and Poultry Bowl, 60
Garlic Turkey Breast with Brussels Sprouts, 61
Chicken with Curry Paste and Coconut Cream, 55
Scallions Chicken Cubes, 61
Tender Chicken and Greens, 56
Chives Chicken, 60
Mozzarella Chicken, 60
Mustard and Garlic Chicken, 58
Chicken with Endives, 58
Mushrooms, Parsley, and Chicken Bowl, 60
Lemon Turkey Bowl, 59
Nutmeg Chicken Cubes, 61
Juicy Rosemary Pork, 66
Scallions Lamb Chops, 73
Rosemary Lamb, 77
Coconut Cream Beef, 76

Parmesan Meat, 65
Autumn Beef Mix, 65
Cheesy Cumin and Garlic Beef, 65
Mint Lamb Cubes, 72
Chili and Chives Lamb, 71
Scallions and Celery Stalk Lamb, 71
Tender Sour Lamb Riblets, 77
Lime Juice Lamb Chops, 81
Parmesan and Scallions Lamb Chops, 74
Rosemary Beef with Swiss Chard, 78
Spring Pork Stew, 67
Chili Lamb with Mushrooms, 78
Spicy Okra and Beef Bowl, 67
Keto Meat with Vegetables, 67
Lamb with Capers, 74
Coriander Meat Stew, 66
Italian Seasoning and Pesto Lamb, 73
Radish and Lamb Stew, 73
Ketogenic Vegetable Recipes, 73
Tomato Passata Kale, 77
Cilantro Brussels Sprouts, 73
Turmeric Bok Choy, 76
Garam Masala Brussels Sprouts, 75
Greens Bowl, 70
Rosemary Sprouts with Avocado, 81
Coconut Cream Bok Choy, 70
Spring Salad, 68
Baby Kale Mix, 68
Broccoli Florets Bowl, 69
Zucchini Cubes Stew, 69
Cumin Swiss Chard with Kalamata Olives, 75
Keto Broccoli Mix, 70
Basil Cream, 70
Baby Spinach Bowl, 81
Broccoli Spread, 75
Garlic Peppers, 75
Sesame and Coriander Kale, 80
Garam Masala Green Cabbage, 75
Garlic Mushroom with Bok Choy, 66
Cabbage and Scallions, 81
sea bass
Lemon Seabass with Avocado, 27
Garlic Sea Bass, 38
Cilantro Sea Bass, 41
Rosemary Sea Bass, 49
Sea Bass and Baby Kale Bowl, 53
shallot
Artichoke and Parmesan Spread, 49
Cumin Pork Chops, 78
Black Olives Salad, 11
Hot Eggs, 18
Meat and Spinach Bowls, 16
Parmesan Eggs Mix, 14
Shallot Salad, 9
Cheese and Turkey Mix, 11
Chives, Spinach, and Shrimps, 11
Chicken Sauce, 19
Spiced Chicken Pan, 19
Parsley Fish Stew, 22
Chili Pepper Soup, 25
Green Beans with Chicken, 15
Coconut Cream Soup, 12
Keto Style Mix, 12
Lemon Seabass with Avocado, 27
Kale Saute, 28

Aromatic Keto Mix, 33
Aromatic Brussel Sprouts, 34
Parmesan Radishes, 34
Cumin Stew, 29
Keto Avocado Bowl, 29
Keto Caps, 35
Ketogenic Seafood and Fish Recipes, 37
Lime Salmon, 38
Tender Lemon Shrimp, 38
Chili Cod, 48
Curry and Garlic Shrimps, 47
Sour Cumin Shrimp, 47
Cod with Coriander Sauce, 47
Tender Duck, 64
Chicken in Tender Sauce, 59
Salsa Verde Turkey, 63
Shredded Cabbage and Chicken Mix, 56
Tender Chicken Cubes with Kalamata Olives, 55
Leek and Turkey, 57
Pork Chops with Vegetables, 71
Pork and Zucchini, 65
Garlic Okra, 81
Rosemary Tomatoes, 68
shrimp
Smoked Shrimp Platter, 39
Scallions and Seafood Salad, 24
Garlic Shrimps Mix, 11
Turmeric Eggs with Shrimps, 20
Seafood and Parsley Bowls, 10
Basil and Shrimps Salad, 12
Chives, Spinach, and Shrimps, 11
Cherry Tomatoes and Shrimps Bowl, 20
Green Onions Shrimp, 25
Cucumbers and Olives Salad, 27
Walnuts Salad, 27
Shrimps and Vegetables, 26
Aromatic Basil Shrimps, 22
Arugula Salad, 27
Vinegar Shrimps, 20
Basil and Seafood Bowls, 16
Kale and Garlic Soup, 16
Keto Style Mix, 12
Lunch Shrimps, 20
Keto Radish Salad, 13
Shrimp and Curry Powder Salsa, 45
Poblano Peppers Dip, 40
Italian Style Shrimps, 45
Seafood Meatballs, 45
Keto Eggs Salad, 43
Dijon Shrimp Skewers, 43
Tender Lemon Shrimp, 38
Scallions Shrimps, 41
Shrimps with Chicken broth, 38
Shrimps with Green Beans, 48
Curry and Garlic Shrimps, 47
Shrimps with Fresh Fennel Bulb, 46
Sour Cumin Shrimp, 47
Shrimps with Endives, 46
Mint and Garlic Shrimp, 54
Coconut Cream Shrimps, 51
Shrimps and Bell Peppers Bowl, 52
Thyme Seafood Bowl, 52
Fennel Seeds Shrimp, 43
Parsley and Shrimps Bowl, 43
Shrimps with Almonds and Parmesan, 48

Recipe Index | 97

Cauli and Shrimps, 48
Shrimps in Sauce, 48
Aromatic Shrimps with Pine Nuts, 50
Marjoram Seafood Bowl, 52
spinach
Scallions and Seafood Salad, 24
Green Avocado Salad, 9
Salmon Salad, 11
Stew Meat Bowls, 14
Seafood and Parsley Bowls, 10
Lime Juice and Poultry Salad, 21
Ginger Smoothie, 10
Micro Greens Bowls, 10
Baby Spinach and Chicken Bowls, 21
Spinach Bowl, 18
Poultry and Cucumber Salad, 18
Baby Spinach and Avocado Salad, 17
Ketogenic Lunch Recipes, 24
Tender Keto Muffins, 25
Bell Peppers Scrambled Eggs, 26
Basil and Shrimps Salad, 12
Chives, Spinach, and Shrimps, 11
Cherry Tomatoes and Shrimps Bowl, 20
Turkey Stew, 22
Capers Mix, 23
Walnuts Salad, 27
Baby Spinach Soup, 21
Crab Mix, 20
Basil and Seafood Bowls, 16
Lunch Shrimps, 20
Soft Meatballs, 12
Mushrooms and Pork, 13
Baby Spinach Saute, 29
Zucchini Medley, 30
Baby Arugula Salad, 32
Green Mushrooms, 32
Green Dip, 41
Coconut Muffins, 44
Greens and Capers Salad, 42
Artichoke and Parmesan Spread, 49
Baby Spinach and Fish Salad, 46
Poultry and Spinach Mix, 63
Poultry Stir Fry, 55
Lemon Turkey Bowl, 59
Meat Salad with Capers, 72
Greens Bowl, 70
Baby Kale Mix, 68
Broccoli Florets Bowl, 69
Walnuts Salad, 74
Baby Spinach Bowl, 81
Red Chili Baby Spinach, 80
stevia
Almonds and Berries Bowls, 9
Vanilla Bowls, 8
Cinnamon Bowls, 8
Keto Cocoa Cream, 87
Stevia Cream, 83
Heavy Cream Mix, 83
Berries Saute, 89
Lime Mousse, 84
Watermelon Soup, 85
Plum and Vanilla Bowls, 84
Mint and Watermelon Salad, 84
Cinnamon Pudding, 86
Berry Pie, 86
Strawberry and Lime Saute, 87

Lime Mix, 87
Cinnamon and Vanilla Balls, 87
Coconut and Lime Zest Custard, 84
Coffee Mousse, 88
Cherries and Ginger Bowls, 85
Cherries and Ginger Bowls, 85
Berry Stew, 85
Sweet and Sour Jam, 89
Vanilla Fudge, 85
strawberries
Sweet Avocado Salad, 10
Almond Pancakes, 17
Almond and Berries Muffins, 89
Vanilla and Berries Bowls, 84
Strawberry and Lime Saute, 87
sunflower seeds
Seeds Snack, 39
Seeds and Nuts Snack, 37
Seeds Mix, 89
T
tomatoes
Green Avocado Salad, 9
Sun Dried Tomatoes and Olives Salsa, 42
Shrimps with Chicken broth, 38
tomatoes (cherry)
Hard Boiled Eggs Bowl, 11
Scallions and Seafood Salad, 24
Salmon Salad, 11
Black Olives Salad, 11
Spiralized Salad, 19
Basil Salad, 21
Oregano and Tuna Casserole, 14
Lime Zest Salad, 9
Shallot Salad, 9
Kale Eggs, 8
Blackberries Salad, 8
Morning Waffles, 25
Baby Spinach and Chicken Bowls, 21
Spinach Bowl, 18
Poultry and Cucumber Salad, 18
Baby Spinach and Avocado Salad, 17
Ketogenic Lunch Recipes, 24
Chicken Pan, 19
Keto Vegetables and Beef Stew, 12
Cherry Tomatoes and Shrimps Bowl, 20
Lime Juice and Chives Salad, 24
Bell Peppers Saute, 26
Parsley Fish Stew, 22
Salmon Stew, 15
Chili Pepper Soup, 25
Chili Powder Meat, 22
Capers Mix, 23
Walnuts Salad, 27
Shrimps and Vegetables, 26
Arugula Salad, 27
Crab Mix, 20
Vinegar Shrimps, 20
Basil and Seafood Bowls, 16
Kale and Garlic Soup, 16
Poultry and Fish Soup, 16
Cabbage Soup, 16
Kalamata and Chicken Salad, 25
Tender Tuna Mix, 13
Aromatic Beef and Greens, 13
Aromatic Keto Mix, 33
Basil Salad, 28

Spring Onions Salad, 28
Dill Mix, 35
Zucchini Medley, 30
Fennel Bulb Salad, 29
Green Chili Pepper Tomatoes, 30
Baby Arugula Salad, 32
Tender Red Cabbage, 32
Jalapeno and Cheddar Cheese Mix, 33
Hemp Seeds Mushrooms, 30
Keto Salsa, 41
Cucumbers Salsa, 39
Peppers Salsa, 39
Greens and Capers Salad, 42
Capers Salsa, 40
Chives Salsa, 42
Chili Cod, 48
Avocado with Cod, 50
Turmeric Calamari, 46
Calamari with Zucchini Zoodles, 46
Tender Sour Tuna, 51
Baby Spinach and Fish Salad, 46
Salmon with Halved Tomatoes, 52
Spicy Chicken Breast Cubes, 60
Coriander Turkey Bowl, 55
Rosemary and Paprika Chicken, 62
Zucchini and Ground Chicken Bowl, 57
Green Beans and Turkey, 58
Poultry Stir Fry, 55
Garlic Cubed Pork, 72
Passata Pork Chops, 77
Pork with Coriander and Shredded Cabbage, 67
Cumin and Chili Powder Lamb Chops, 76
Keto Lamb Bowl, 71
Spring Pork Stew, 67
Coriander Meat Stew, 66
Tender Beef Roast, 73
Italian Seasoning and Pesto Lamb, 73
Meat Salad with Capers, 72
Rosemary Tomatoes, 68
Spring Salad, 68
Cilantro Avocado, 68
Cherry Tomatoes and Greens Salad, 69
Chard Bowl, 82
Walnuts Salad, 74
Basil Cream, 70
Cabbage and Scallions, 81
trout
Turmeric Trout, 37
Dijon Mustard Trout, 41
Aromatic Trout, 52
Red Pepper Flakes Trout, 48
Trout Bowl, 49
tuna
Oregano and Tuna Casserole, 14
Capers and Tuna Salad, 18
Capers Mix, 23
Tender Tuna Mix, 13
Tuna with Vegetables, 50
Basil Tuna and Cayenne Pepper Bowl, 46
Perfect Keto Tuna, 51
Tender Sour Tuna, 51
Ginger Tuna, 43
Baby Spinach and Fish Salad, 46
Balsamic Tuna with Spring Onions, 44
Spiced Tuna Fillets, 53

turkey
- Onion Powder Eggs, 18
- Lime Juice and Poultry Salad, 21
- Cheese and Turkey Mix, 11
- Lime Juice and Chives Salad, 24
- Turkey Stew, 22
- Poultry Stew, 22
- Curry Turkey, 22
- Turkey and Endives, 13
- Oregano Turkey, 56
- Chili Powder Turkey, 63
- Broccoli and Poultry Bowl, 60
- Garlic Turkey Breast with Brussels Sprouts, 61
- Coriander Turkey Bowl, 55
- Greens and Turkey Bowl, 62
- Salsa Verde Turkey, 63
- Leek and Turkey, 57
- Red Chili Pepper Turkey, 56
- Fragrant Cumin Turkey, 63
- Tender Turkey in Sauce, 62
- Mustard Powder Turkey, 64
- Poultry and Spinach Mix, 63
- Poultry Bake, 62
- Poultry Stir Fry, 55
- Bella Mushrooms and Turkey, 59
- Lemon Turkey Bowl, 59
- Aromatic Spiced Turkey, 61

W
walnuts
- Stevia and Nuts Bowls, 8
- Mix of Seeds Bowls, 26
- Spinach Bowl, 18
- Walnuts Salad, 27
- Arugula Salad, 27
- Walnuts and Beef Bowl, 17
- Turkey and Endives, 13
- Classic Keto Bowl, 31
- Walnuts Dip, 38
- Seeds Snack, 39
- Chia and Flaxseeds Muffins, 47
- Nuts Bowls, 10
- Walnuts Snack Bowls, 38
- Lime Salmon, 38
- Nutmeg Salmon Bowl, 44
- Tender Sour Lamb Riblets, 77
- Cherry Tomatoes and Greens Salad, 69
- Walnuts Salad, 74
- Stevia Cream, 83
- Walnuts and Avocado Bowls, 84
- Swerve and Watermelon Mix, 83

watermelon
- Watermelon Soup, 85
- Mint and Watermelon Salad, 84
- Swerve and Watermelon Mix, 83
- Watermelon Custard, 86

Z
zucchini
- Cilantro and Eggs Mix, 14
- Allspice Zucchini, 24
- Almond and Vegetables Muffins, 24
- Cheddar Cheese Bake, 18
- Spiced Chicken Pan, 19
- Meat Casserole, 15
- Aromatic Basil Shrimps, 22
- Spiced Meat Stew, 16
- Keto Style Mix, 12
- Zucchini Medley, 30
- Dill Zoodles, 29
- Sage Zucchini, 30
- Cajun Seasonings and Keto Vegetables, 36
- Caraway Seeds Mix of Vegetables, 36
- Tender Zucchini Rice, 31
- Paprika Zucchini Chips, 41
- Nutmeg Platter, 40
- Mozzarella and Vegetables Dip, 37
- Tuna with Vegetables, 50
- Basil Tuna and Cayenne Pepper Bowl, 46
- Coriander Turkey Bowl, 55
- Zucchini and Ground Chicken Bowl, 57
- Poultry Stir Fry, 55
- Spring Pork Stew, 67
- Zucchini Cubes Stew, 69
- Chard Bowl, 82
- Coconut Cream Zucchini, 70
- Zucchini Mousse, 88
- Spiralized Salad, 19
- Turmeric Pancakes, 17
- Garlic Zucchini, 17
- Keto Cheese Mix, 15
- Scallions Zucchini, 28
- Pesto and Zucchini Dip, 38
- Calamari with Zucchini Zoodles, 46
- Pork and Zucchini, 65
- Vinegar Beef, 72
- Turmeric Sliced Zucchini Mix, 74
- Dill Mix, 79

Made in United States
North Haven, CT
18 February 2022